Ellen Henrietta (Swallow) Richards

Food Materials and Their Adulterations

Ellen Henrietta (Swallow) Richards

Food Materials and Their Adulterations

ISBN/EAN: 9783744645942

Printed in Europe, USA, Canada, Australia, Japan

Cover: Foto ©Andreas Hilbeck / pixelio.de

More available books at **www.hansebooks.com**

FOOD MATERIALS

AND

THEIR ADULTERATIONS.

BY

ELLEN H. RICHARDS,

INSTRUCTOR IN SANITARY CHEMISTRY IN THE MASSACHUSETTS
INSTITUTE OF TECHNOLOGY.

AUTHOR OF "CHEMISTRY OF COOKING AND CLEANING."

NEW AND CORRECTED EDITION.

BOSTON:
HOME SCIENCE PUBLISHING CO.
1898.

FIRST EDITION.
Copyright, 1885,
By Estes and Lauriat.

SECOND EDITION.
Copyright, 1898,
By Home Science Publishing Co.

PRESS OF
Rockwell and Churchill
BOSTON

PREFACE.

THERE is neither novelty in the information which this little volume seeks to convey, nor originality in the manner of presenting it; but when its preparation was begun, some years since, the facts here considered were for the most part found scattered through large and costly technical works, written for the conditions existing in England and Germany. The books claiming to be popular expositions were either so old as to be out of date, were sensational, or otherwise unsatisfactory.

One excellent English work has recently appeared which is so suitable and admirable in form, as well as in material, that at the first glance it seemed superfluous to issue the present one. Yet Church's "Food" was prepared especially for the visitors to the Bethnal Green branch of the South Kensington Museum, London, while the place which this little volume is intended to fill is that of giving useful information in a form available and attractive for schools and for home reading, without technicalities or unnecessary details. It has been compiled from many sources, and it would be impossible to credit each book with the special facts derived from it, since the same thing in different forms is often found in several works. Quotation marks are intended to indicate all passages taken verbatim. The names of the books consulted will be found in the list at the end of the volume. It is in the hope that these works may be more widely known, and the subjects of which they treat more earnestly studied, that this slight contribution is sent forth.

The conclusions are a result of ten years' experience in laboratory examination of food materials.

The author is especially indebted to Miss S. MINNS and to Miss L. M. PEABODY for valuable aid, both in the laboratory and in the preparation of the text.

BOSTON, *December*, 1885.

CONTENTS.

I.	THE RELATION OF GENERAL INTELLIGENCE TO THE QUALITY OF THE FOOD SUPPLY . . .	7
II.	WATER, TEA, COFFEE, COCOA	24
III.	CEREAL FOODS.— BARLEY, RICE, OATS, MAIZE, RYE, AND WHEAT	70
IV.	MILK, BUTTER, CHEESE	88
V.	SUGAR.	97
VI.	CANNED FRUITS AND MEATS, OR TINNED GOODS	118
VII.	CONDIMENTS.	125
VIII.	PERISHABLE FOODS, AND THE MEANS FOR PRESERVING THEM.— MEAT, FRUIT, ETC. . . .	144
IX.	OTHER MATERIALS USED IN COOKING	151
X.	PRINCIPLES OF DIET	162

LIST OF WORKS CONSULTED 177
INDEX 181

FOOD MATERIALS

AND

THEIR ADULTERATIONS.

I.

THE RELATION OF GENERAL INTELLIGENCE TO THE QUALITY OF THE FOOD SUPPLY.

THE prosperity of a nation depends upon the health and the morals of its citizens; and the health and the morals of a people depend mainly upon the food they eat, and the homes they live in.

Strong men and women cannot be "raised" on insufficient food. Good-tempered, temperate, highly moral men cannot be expected from a race which eats badly cooked food, irritating to the digestive organs and unsatisfying to the appetite. Wholesome and palatable food is the first step in good morals, and is conducive to ability in business, skill in trade, and healthy tone in literature.

This being granted, what office is of more importance to the State than that of the provider of food for the families composing it? Indeed, some of the younger States of the Union have recognized the two fundamental professions upon which their prosperity rests, and have established in their agricultural colleges a parallel course of domestic economy to complete the education of the girls.

This is an instance of wisdom, an example which our Eastern States might well copy; for not only in the homes on the Western plains, but in all our towns and villages, do the housewives need to know something of the materials of daily consumption.

The conditions of life have changed here in New England so rapidly and completely, that our young housewives find themselves very much at a loss. The methods of their mothers and grandmothers will no longer answer. *They* had no trouble with their soap, for they superintended its making and knew its properties. *They* knew how colored fabrics should be washed, for they had the coloring done under their own eyes. *We* buy everything, and have no idea of the processes by which the articles are produced, and have no means of knowing beforehand what the quality may be. Relatively, we are in a state of barbarous ignorance, as compared with our grandmothers, about the common articles of daily use.

The last fifty years have seen such a marvellous advance in applied science, especially in applied chemistry, that it is no wonder that housewives have fallen somewhat behind ; but it is high time for them to awake to the importance of their profession. Unscrupulous manufacturers call in the aid of the chemist's art to enable them to deceive the credulous "lady of the house," and the only remedy is for "the lady" to acquire knowledge which will enable her to detect such palpable frauds as are daily practised.

Modern invention and modern extravagance have so complicated modern housekeeping, that there is little wonder that the untrained mistress and the untrained servant together often make an abode of ill-temper, of constant warfare and change, of discomfort and danger to all its inmates, instead of a restful family fireside where all the troubles and vexations of the outside world should be shut out, and where ruffled tempers should sweeten, and the best intellect expand. Our housekeeping has become so complicated and laborious that it cannot go on indefinitely in this way;

there must soon come a crash unless some way can be devised for a quiet revolution.

This is an age of progress. We cannot go back to any example in the past. Educated women must mark out a new plan for themselves. Our girls must be taught to recognize the profession of housekeeping as one of the highest, although not necessarily the only one; but whatever art or accomplishment they may acquire besides, let them consider that the management of a household is not to be neglected. The properly educated housekeeper is not a drudge: she has all the forces of nature at her command, — the lightning harnessed to give her light; the stored-up energy of past ages at her command by the turning of a stopcock; swift steamships and railways bring to her fruits and vegetables from all climes; the vast prairies furnish meat, game, and flour; mechanical skill gives her all kinds of labor-saving devices; the general prosperity and improving taste of the country admit of tasteful decoration of the rooms. Surely, never did housekeeping present so many charms. Alas! the winged Pegasus is too strong for his unskilled rider, for in his train has come a style of living both extravagant and demoralizing. All this delicate machinery and costly luxury are committed by ignorant mistresses to still more ignorant servants,— conservative by inheritance and superstitious by nature, restless with the very air of the new, and to them wonderful country, where all men are equal, and naturally bewildered by the novelties of the new life, so different from their simple one. What wonder that the complicated machinery comes to grief, and the tempers of both mistress and maid are spoiled in attempting the impossible!

The only remedy is for our girls to learn something practical about these forces, and the nature of the materials which are scattered about so freely. The distinction between an educated cook and an uneducated one of the same skill is, that the educated one can tell some one else just how and why she takes each step, while the uneducated one can do the thing, but cannot tell any one else how or why she does it. Let our school-girls bear this in mind, and so study their chemistry and physics that they can tell why this and that should, or should not be done. A little actual knowledge wonderfully simplifies things, and adds interest to the commonest deeds.

Our housekeeping is brought down from its high estate by being left to persons born and reared under such totally different conditions that they cannot understand the complications of our way of living. Too much is expected of them, and they are soon spoiled and rendered unfit for service, or for caring for homes for themselves. A little care, patience, and instruction would save the majority of them, and make a vast difference in the homes of the land.

Within the memory of the present generation there has crept into the heads of the great American people a most pernicious and insidious idea, — that labor with the hands alone is degrading and beneath the dignity of a free American citizen. Nowhere has this been more noticeable than in the place to which housework has been relegated.

To judge by the opinion of the average school-girl, one would think that housekeeping required no more thought than the breaking of stones on the highway. Such may listen with profit to Ruskin when he says: "It is a no less fatal error to despise labor when regulated by intellect than to value it for its own sake. In these days we are always trying to separate the two. We want one man to be always thinking, another to be always working; and we call the one a gentleman, and the other an operative, whereas the workman ought often to be thinking and the thinker to be working, and both should be gentlemen in the best sense. Now it is only by labor that thought can be made healthy, and only by thought that labor can be made happy."

If this is assented to, then is not the conclusion clear, that, if our girls were capable of thinking about the many problems of housework, and of investigating new and better ways, they would find the work an interesting and worthy one?

It is only in the undeveloped stages of a mechanical invention that it is complicated and runs with friction. The perfected machine is noiseless in its action, and simple in its construction. The machinery of daily life should respond to the slightest touch of the house engineer, the one who knows all about it. The running of a household is a no less responsible task than the running of a steamboat or an engine.

The time has come when the same kind of care must be given to the food of the family as the stock-raiser gives to that of his animals. The modern stock farm has given us most of the scientific knowledge we possess on the question of foods. All this because it pays to know the composition of the food, etc. Shall the human animal be considered of less consequence?

It is a wonder that political economists do not take up this subject, for the ultimate welfare of the country depends upon securing the maximum of utility for the money spent. The money's worth must be obtained from both material and labor. The law of utility requires an adequate return for the value consumed. A loaf of bread eaten by a farm-hand returns more than its value in the produce of that man's labor; so it should be with all labor, whether mechanical or literary. A loaf of bread allowed to mould brings no return in wheat or in useful thought, and it is therefore wasted, — so much value thrown away. So, too, if a family consume at one meal three times as much food as is needed to keep them in perfect health, the excess is wasted, and sometimes worse, in that it causes disease. Not that a family which can afford beef should live on corn meal, but that if the food is not wisely used for pleasure or nourishment, it is wasted.

The time has come when we must have a science of domestic economy, and it must be worked out in the homes of our educated women. The conditions of life are so peculiar in this country that no plan made for another land will suit us, and we must make our own. A knowledge of the elements of chemistry and physics must be applied to the daily living.

It is not merely to the heads of large and expensive families that the simple knowledge is of use. In the address of the President of the American Institute of Mining Engineers, in August, 1882, we find the following pertinent remarks: "If technical instruction and skill in our workmen be essential to the economical development of industry, and the welfare of those engaged in it, the technical education of their wives is not one whit less important. Those who are familiar with the expenditures and mode of life of the wage classes at our chief mining and metallurgical centres cannot fail to be struck by the amount of waste and the extravagance of their expenditures. I do not mean to have you infer that they live too well, but that through ignorance of the actual and comparative values of different edibles, through ignorance of the best ways of preparing palatable food, of housekeeping in all its branches, it is not uncommon to find a mining family spending more for a wretched living and uncomfortable home than is spent in many a pleasant and comparatively luxurious one. We are all but too familiar with strikes against greater or less reductions, or for increase of wages; but the working classes have more to gain in comfort and well-being by the better technical education of their wives and daughters, by more intelligence and skill in their homes, than they could gain should they obtain the most extravagant demands for which a strike was ever instituted. Scientific housekeeping is neither beneath the attention of the refined, nor beyond the reach of the uncultured. It is the duty of the rich: it is the salvation of the poor."

A great deal may be done by economy in the preparation of food, and in the substitution of one kind for another, according to the cost at different seasons of the year. Here a knowledge of the composition of the various articles of diet will enable one to choose, and yet to give the family all the constituents needed. Tables of the relative value of foods such as those in Bulletin 28, U. S. Dept. of Agriculture, 1896, will guide a wise housekeeper in her selection.

Few people realize the value of cornmeal as an article of diet. It is given on good authority that a young woman, who was temporarily reduced to the closest straits in a pecuniary point of view, in order to save most of her small salary for dependent relatives, lived on corn meal cooked in various ways for a whole year, with only a dinner every Sunday at a friend's house. She kept well and hearty on a peck of Indian meal a month; so that her whole living cost only about ten dollars for the year, as she prepared it herself. This young woman knew how to prepare her food so that it was palatable; and it was much better than the tea, slops, and baker's bread, with which so many working-women try to sustain life.

It seems a great waste to spend twenty hours a week in making pies, cakes, and puddings for a family of five persons, at a cost of five dollars for the raw material, when the raw or cooked fruit for dessert can be obtained for three dollars a week, and the time of preparation as well as the fuel be saved. Many families who now keep two maids could live just as comfortably with one, if the mistress could plan the work in all these labor-saving ways.

Cooking-schools and classes are doing good work in their line, and they should be introduced very much more widely; but instruction must go farther, and include sanitary principles and the branches of domestic economy. We very much need this sort of instruction introduced into our schools in such form that the practical application will go into the homes.

One of the most puzzling problems which a modern housewife has to solve, is to learn the quality of the various food materials which she provides for the use of the family, and to know how to apportion them. So much has been said on the subject of adulteration in the past few years, that the peace of mind of a conscientious woman is quite gone, and she appeals to the law-makers to protect her family.

It has been the history of every harmful adulteration, that, as soon as the public became aware of the nature of it, its manufacture was stopped, and some new device substituted. The remedy, then, for this sort of fraud, is the education of the general public to such an extent that they can, with some degree of probability, detect any flagrant case of adulteration or substitution. It is the aim of this little work to place in the hands of housekeepers such information as will enable them to purchase intelligently, and to know in what direction to be suspicious. The nature of the adulterations will vary from year to year with the advance of knowledge, and with the detection and exposure of the accustomed frauds; so a careful watch is needed to keep the dealers and manufacturers in check.

Dr. Hassall, in his classic work on food and its adulterations, says that from 1850 to 1856 he examined three thousand samples of the principal articles of consumption, and found that few which could be profitably adulterated were not so; from that time to 1875 he found less adulteration, partly due to the exposures made, partly to stricter legal enactments, and partly because detection is now more certain. It seemed to him in 1875 as if frauds were again on the increase.

Demand is the great cause of supply; and if many of the reasons for complaint were examined, it would be found that the grocers, of whom we so bitterly complain, are only supplying the demand of their customers. Few dealers are in a position to instruct their customers; there are occasional philanthropists among them, but most of them must make money, and they can do this only by supplying what the public want; the superstition yet lingering in the minds of people is nowhere shown more clearly than in the purchases they make for every-day use. The credulity with which the average housekeeper swallows the statements of the unscrupulous advertiser is worthy of the Middle Ages. Science, and especially chemical science, has achieved so many marvellous triumphs within the last fifty years, that it is looked upon as an occult knowledge, having the power which was attributed to the alchemy of the Middle Ages; and even intelligent persons, perhaps unconsciously, look upon chemical operations as capable of transforming substances in as subtle a manner as was claimed to be possible by the old-time searcher after the philosopher's stone. As a result, the average housekeeper is a fit subject for the modern alchemist, — the man who can turn sal-soda or whiting into gold by a few neatly turned phrases calculated to impress the housewife with the profound wisdom of the manufacturer.

In considering the probabilities of adulteration, one important fact must not be overlooked. When prices are low and food is plentiful, there is much less reason for admixture of foreign substances; but when prices are high and any article scarce, then is adulteration rife. Take, for example, cream of tartar: in ordinary years, when money is plentiful and gold at par, it can be bought at from thirty-five to forty cents a pound;

but when gold was two dollars or more, as during the war, and when the risk of importation became considerable, cream of tartar sold for two dollars or so a pound. The poor people could not pay fifty cents for what they had been accustomed to get for ten; but they did not know enough of the principles of cooking to get along without it, and so they asked for something cheaper. During those years there was very little of the genuine article sold under the name, and the result was poor bread and injured health.

A very good example of the law of supply and demand was given to the writer by a man of strict integrity, but a man of business, who understood the public temper. When quite young he kept a small grocery store in one of the suburbs of Boston. Cream of tartar had just come into use. A woman who had been in the habit of purchasing her supplies at a neighboring grocery came to him one day for some articles. The young man prided himself on the good quality of his goods, therefore felt quite sure she would be pleased, and give him her custom. What was his surprise to have her come back and complain of the quality of his cream of tartar. It did not make as good bread as that which she had been buying. He ventured to suggest that perhaps it was strong, and that she used too much; but she would not be satisfied, and wanted another kind, so he made up a package for her of two thirds cream of tartar and one third rice flour; this satisfied her, and she became his customer.

The same story has been told repeatedly of milk. People complained of the yellow, and wished for the blue milk, such as they had been using. All this is a great temptation; and we can hardly expect our grocers to become philanthropists and teachers of the people. Their business is to supply the public with the articles which it demands, and it is from education of the public that we must look for redress. There is great danger to the moral sense of the community from this sort of cheating, — this obtaining money under false pretences (for it is nothing else). And the public is content to be cheated; it should be aroused, and by a knowledge of food materials a stop may be put to most frauds.

The unanimous testimony of all chemists who have carefully investigated the extent to which adulteration of food is carried on in the United States is, that, while there exists adulteration injurious to health, there is a much greater injury to the morals of the community, and loss to the pockets of the people. In other words, the point to which public attention should be mainly directed is the question of paying a high price for an inferior article. In some portions of the country ground gypsum — at perhaps a cent a pound — is sold for cream of tartar at ten cents a quarter of a pound ; now this fraud can be detected by any one who knows that cream of tartar is soluble in hot water, while gypsum is not. A cupful of boiling water poured upon half a teaspoonful of good cream of tartar will dissolve it almost instantly, giving a nearly transparent liquid.

Some simple tests will be found in the following pages, and it is hoped that some little enlightenment may result. A knowledge of the elementary principles of chemistry, as much at least as is given in the "Chemistry of Cooking and Cleaning," is desirable ; and if a little qualitative practice can be added, the explanations will be clearer. For girls in the high schools, furnished with laboratories, the tests will be very simple. References will be given to works where further information may be obtained.

II.

WATER, TEA, COFFEE, COCOA.

IN importance to health second only to pure air is the quality of the water drunk. It may be even considered as a food, for there is at least a probability that its office in the system is more than that of a regulator of temperature and a diluent of the blood. From a sanitary point of view, next in importance to the quality of the water used is that of the other liquids which are more and more frequently substituted for it, namely, tea, coffee, and cocoa. Beer and wine are neither foods nor necessary beverages in this land of good water and cheap coffee, hence they are not here considered.

WATER.

This section is composed of extracts taken, by permission, from "Water Supply, Chemical and Sanitary," by William Ripley Nichols.

Drinking Water and Disease.

With reference to their use for town and household supply, we shall roughly divide all natural waters into four classes, as follows: —

1. Rain water;
2. Surface water, including streams and lakes;
3. Ground water, including shallow wells;
4. Deep-seated water, including deep wells, artesian wells, and springs.

Under each of these heads we shall study the advantages and disadvantages of the particular class of water, the liability of pollution, etc.; but first we will consider, in a general way, the connection which exists, or is supposed by some to exist, between drinking water and disease.

A water containing a considerable amount of dissolved substances, — one which could properly be denominated a mineral water, — would not be thought of for a public water supply; and would seldom be used as a regular beverage except for the sake of real or fancied medicinal effect; a small amount, however, of mineral matter is generally considered an advantage. The presence of the substances which ordinarily exist in solution in natural waters must not be regarded as necessary, because on shipboard experience has shown that distilled water, properly aerated, is perfectly wholesome. It appears that distilled water, soft surface water, and moderately hard spring or well water are all wholesome, and may be drunk without inconvenience by persons accustomed to their use. It is, however, true that a person who is in the habit of drinking a soft water generally experiences some derangement of the digestive organs on beginning to use hard water, and *vice versa*. It is contended by some that the human system needs salts of lime, etc., that these compounds are furnished in an assimilable form in water, and that, consequently, a somewhat hard water is more advantageous for town supply. Statistics have been brought together to support this view by comparing the death rate of various towns with the hardness of the water supply; but the death rate depends upon too many factors to be used as the chief argument in this connection. It is, however, the result of general observation, that a hard water of which the hardness is due to salts of magnesia or to sulphate of lime is not well suited for drinking, and is injurious to most persons.

A hard water is, generally speaking, one which contains compounds of lime or magnesia in solution.

Waters, especially surface waters, containing much vegetable matter are also, in some cases, unwholesome. The water of marshes is sometimes the cause of diarrhœa and other diseases of this character, and is supposed by some to cause malarial fevers. The mere presence of vegetable organic matter, however, is not sufficient to produce these effects, because many waters which are quite deeply colored by vegetable matter are proved by experience to be perfectly wholesome.

While some waters are thus in their natural condition unwholesome, and may be the cause of sickness, the attention of sanitarians and water experts is directed nowadays principally to the effect of water which is polluted by the waste materials from manufactories and dwellings, or by the sewage of towns and cities; and it is generally held, especially in England and the United States, that water thus polluted may be, and frequently is, the cause of certain specific diseases. Before discussing this question directly, it is important to have a general idea of the present prevailing view with reference to the so-called zymotic diseases, and to understand what is meant by the "germ theory."

Many clear liquids containing organic matter of animal or vegetable origin, — such, for instance, as infusions of hay, infusion of turnip, urine, etc., — if exposed to the air, gradually become turbid or cloudy; or perhaps a film forms on the surface of the liquid, or a deposit upon the walls of the vessel which contains it. The cause of the turbidity is shown by the microscope to be the presence of countless minute organized bodies, — some rod-like, others globular, — which prove to be capable of self-propagation, and which are endowed with motion, at least under certain conditions. Similar organisms are found in the "dust" which floats in the air, and which may be collected by causing a current of air to impinge upon a surface moistened with glycerine; they occur in rain water, particularly in that which falls in the beginning of a shower, in surface waters, and elsewhere. They are found especially where there is decomposing organic matter, and perform an active part in promoting or producing the chemical changes which take place. In certain diseases of men and of the lower animals, organisms which, in their general character, are similar to those thus described, have been found in the blood or in the substance of various organs, and their connection with the disease seems to be something more than a coincidence; there seems, indeed, to be a casual connection.

The "Germ Theory" of disease is, that many diseases are due to the presence and propagation in the system of these minute organisms, which are popularly spoken of under the general name Bacteria, under which term are included also organisms which, as far as known, are harmless.

Dr. Sternberg, the Surgeon-General of the United States Army, in a recent address said: "The generalization that all infectious diseases are due to the introduction into the bodies of susceptible individuals of living germs capable of reproduction is based upon exact knowledge, gained chiefly during the past twenty years, as regards the specific infectious agents or germs of a considerable number of the diseases of this class."

Admitting the necessary presence of these minute organisms in the bodies of persons sick with infectious or other germ diseases, organisms which, at least in certain stages of their development, can exist outside the human body and retain their vitality for a long time, the question arises how they can find their way into the systems of healthy persons to produce disease. The two most obvious of the possible carriers of disease are the air we breathe and the water we drink. We have no difficulty in supposing that emanations from sick persons may find their way into the air, and especially in the form of dry dust may be borne long distances; moreover, the dejections of the sick and the water in which their clothes or their persons have been washed may often reach wells or other sources of drinking-water. Of the diseases which are supposed to be caused by these microorganisms, to be propagated by germs, those which have been, with the greatest unanimity, ascribed to the use of impure drinking-water are typhoid fever and cholera.

Although it cannot be asserted that drinking-water is the only means by which the zymotic diseases may be propagated, the coincidences, however, if coin-

NOTE. — The years which have passed since this chapter was written have only confirmed the belief that drinking-water is often a carrier of disease, and that typhoid fever is usually waterborne, except when carried by milk; that it is not contagious or communicated from one person to another except by close and careless contact. So sure have sanitary authorities become on this point that water from running streams which receive sewage is not considered safe for drinking or culinary purposes, unless biologically filtered.

cidences they be, are most remarkable, and every year adds to their number.

There are many instances where the closing of the suspected source of supply has at once put a stop to the further spread of the disease; there are also instances where people have assembled in numbers on account of some celebration, and sickness has followed in the case of a large proportion of those who have used a certain water, while the others have not been affected; latterly there have been cases where sickness has broken out among families obtaining their milk from the same source, and investigation has shown that impure water was used in the dairy.

As this is a matter which, in the present state of science, cannot be absolutely proved or disproved, the duty of those who have to advise or to decide in matters relating to water supply is perfectly clear: it is to err on the side of safety, to admit the hypothesis that specific diseases may be conveyed by the drinking water, and to guard all sources of domestic and public supply from the possibility of contamination by the dejections of persons sick with zymotic diseases and by excremental matter generally.

Although there are many substances of vegetable

origin which are violent poisons, such as the vegetable alkaloids, for example, it is generally held that refuse of vegetable origin is of much less importance as a source of pollution than that coming from animal sources. This is probably true in general, but it is well known that the vegetable refuse from certain manufacturing operations may be very offensive; such, for instance, is the refuse from starch factories, the water in which flax has been retted, etc. That such water would be unfit to drink, unless enormously diluted, one can hardly doubt.

However views may differ as to the possible injury from this or that particular form of contamination, we are safe in accepting the two following principles as fundamental guides in the selection of a water for a water supply: —

1. A water suitable for domestic supply must be free from all substances which are known to produce an injurious effect on the human system, or which are suspected with good reason or on good authority to produce such an effect.

2. The water should be, as far as practicable, free from all substances and from all associations which offend the general æsthetic sense of the community,

and thus affect the system through the imagination, even if there is good reason to suppose that it is in itself perfectly harmless.

Again, most persons naturally object to water as muddy as that of most of our Western streams, in spite of the favorable testimony of those in the habit of using it; but by a short residence in St. Louis, for instance, most persons soon become accustomed to the turbidity. The turbidity is a real objection to the water; but in the case of a water like that of the Missouri, a town would not be justified in postponing the introduction of the water because it was not able at the same time to adopt a scheme for its thorough filtration. In the same way, if the only objection to a river or pond water is a yellow or brownish-yellow color derived from vegetable, especially peaty matter, the water need not be condemned, although most persons would prefer a colorless water.

Undoubtedly the best water for drinking is a moderately soft spring water, in which all possibility of contamination is out of the question. Unfortunately, however, it is comparatively seldom that such water is available in quantities sufficient for the supply of large towns. Many spring waters are so hard that, while not unsuited for drinking, they are unsuited for many manufacturing uses, for use in steam boilers, and for washing and culinary purposes.

It is a mistake to claim that the water which is absolutely best for drinking must be chosen at any expense as a town supply : when a soft surface water free from appreciable pollution can be obtained, it entails a very serious and constant expense to reject it in favor of a hard water, which may, to be sure, be clearer to the eye and somewhat more pleasant to the taste. There are surface waters and there are surface-water supplies which are undoubtedly bad ; but a good surface water, such as may be taken directly from many streams, or such as may be obtained from deep lakes and from proper storage basins, is perfectly well suited for domestic use or for town supply. There are some who maintain an opinion contrary to that which has been expressed. The Vienna Commission, in 1864, rejected surface waters from among the waters suitable for domestic use, on the ground of their variable temperature and their liability to pollution. The German Public Health Association, at the Dantzic meeting in 1880, by a small majority and after a lively discussion, adopted a resolution to the effect that spring water or properly protected ground water was the only admissible source of supply; but two years later this dictum was modified so as to include filtered river water as fulfilling the required conditions, and this conclusion is sanctioned by practice and experience.

The Pollution of Domestic Wells.

In isolated dwellings and in villages and small towns not yet provided with a public water supply, drinking water must, as a rule, be obtained either by collecting the rain water and storing it in tanks and cisterns, or else by sinking wells. On account of the clearness and nearly uniform temperature of the ground water, the latter method is usually preferred when practicable. In the majority of cases the location of the well is dictated simply by convenience, and it frequently happens that it is in close proximity to a privy, or to cesspools, or to a barn or stable. The result is that the well is very liable to pollution, and, more often than not, it is simply a question of time when the water shall become unfit for use.

The pollution of the well generally takes place gradually. The ground gradually becomes charged with the soakage from the privies and manure heaps, and percolating rain water carries the impure matter into the ground water from which the well draws its supply. In other cases, actual channels are formed, by which the foul liquid trickles or flows into the well itself, or a leaky drain, laid near the well, may be the source of the trouble.

Whatever views may be held of the effect upon the human system of drinking such water, there is no question whatever as to the pollution itself; and although the water may appear clear and bright, and be inoffensive to the senses, chemical examination may show that it is highly charged with the products of decomposition. Moreover, there are hundreds of cases on record where sickness has been coincident with the use of polluted well water, and although the evidence is of necessity circumstantial, it is too striking to be disregarded. In the present state of knowledge, it must be said that the continued use of well water proved to be polluted is as unjustifiable as suicide generally is. Under what conditions the water may become injurious, and when, no one can say.

Household Filtration.

In localities where there is a public water supply, it is without doubt the duty of the water board or company to deliver the water to consumers in a condition fit for domestic use. If the source which is, on the whole, the most available for the water supply is such that filtration is absolutely necessary, the water should be filtered on the large scale by the authority controlling the works. Practically, however, in the case of most existing water supplies the water as delivered to the consumers may be appreciably improved by filtration; household filtration is also often necessary in country residences and in the smaller towns where there is no public supply, and where it is necessary to use rain water which has been stored in tanks or cisterns. For filtration on the household scale, numerous devices have been made and patented, and the greatest variety of material has been proposed.

Many sorts of porous stone, sand, powdered glass, bricks, iron in turnings and other forms, vegetable and animal charcoal, sponge, wool, flannel, cotton, straw, sawdust, excelsior, and wire-gauze, — these are some of the substances which are used. A filter suitable for household use must be made of a material which cannot communicate any injurious or offensive quality to the water which passes through it; it must remove from the water all suspended particles, so as to render the water bright and clear; and it must either be readily cleaned, or the filtering material must be such as to be readily renewed. In addition to these requirements, it is of great advantage if the filter is able to remove a noticeable amount of the dissolved organic matter which most waters contain.

As to the filtering material, the author is satisfied that there is nothing, on the whole, better than well-burned animal charcoal (bone-coal). This material, as is well known, possesses great power in removing organic matter from solution, and is used in the arts to decolorize colored solutions: on many organic substances it acts, not simply by adhesion, but apparently by bringing them into contact with oxygen, and thus absolutely destroying them. Its power does not last indefinitely, and a bone-coal filter, like a filter of any other material, requires cleansing and renewal at proper intervals. Other materials to be mentioned render good service, and in certain sorts of filters, as for instance those made for attachment to ordinary cocks or faucets, the bone-coal possesses no essential advantage.

The Softening of Hard Water.

The hardness of water is generally due to the presence of compounds of lime or magnesia. While a moderately hard water may be perfectly well suited for drinking, for almost all the other purposes of a water supply a soft water is preferable, other things being equal. If common soap be added to hard water the water seems to curdle, but no permanent froth or lather is formed until, by the mutual action of the soap and the compounds of lime and magnesia on each other, the latter are completely converted into a lime or magnesia soap, — an insoluble substance which forms the curd alluded to. After this point is reached, any additional soap becomes available for washing, but the curdy water is less efficient as a detergent. Hard water is as a rule much less desirable for culinary purposes than soft water. Finally, hard water is also objectionable on account of the "scale" which forms in steam boilers in which it is used; in manufacturing towns this becomes a matter of great importance.

Permanent Hardness.

The permanent hardness is usually caused by the presence of the sulphates (or other soluble salts) of lime and magnesia, gypsum (sulphate of lime) being the most common; the action on soap is the same as that of the bicarbonates, which cause temporary hardness. Water containing sulphate of lime may be softened by adding carbonate of soda, and this is the method commonly employed in the laundry. The chemistry of the process is this: when carbonate of soda in solution is mixed with sulphate of lime in solution, there are formed carbonate of lime (which settles out in the solid form) and sulphate of soda (which remains dissolved); a similar action takes place with other soluble compounds of lime and magnesia.

The expense of this treatment makes it impracticable to soften in this way the entire water supply of a town, a large portion of which is used for purposes where the hardness of the water is a matter of indifference. Sulphate of lime becomes insoluble in water at high temperatures and contributes to the formation of scale in steam boilers; hence, for technical purposes it is desirable to remove the sulphate, and the process just indicated, or some other method, may be employed to advantage.

The most simple manner of treating a water known or suspected to be impure is to boil it, although it is by no means certain that immunity from harm is thus in all cases assured. There is, however, evidence to show the value of the treatment. If after the boiling the water is iced, it becomes, of course, more palatable. It is stated that the Chinese and Japanese drink no water that has not been boiled; and when we consider the unsanitary conditions which exist in those countries and the character of the water used, it seems as if boiling the water must prevent ills that would otherwise befall the people.

Service Pipes.

The service pipes for house distribution in connection with a public water supply are generally of lead, this metal being employed on account of the facility with which it may be worked. Lead pipes are also sometimes used for conveying well or spring water to individual residences. Various waters act very differently upon lead, — some corroding it rapidly, others only to a very slight extent under similar circumstances.

The cause of the corrosion is to be sought in the dissolved oxygen, of which all waters contain more or less, and in certain saline substances, the presence of which determines a more violent action. It is generally felt, for instance, that the presence of nitrates, nitrites, and ammoniacal salts increases the action of water on lead, while carbonates, sulphates, and notably phosphates, hinder such action; but while certain general statements may be truthfully made as the result of laboratory experiment and from the analysis of waters whose action on lead has been learned by experience, it is a rather hazardous thing for a chemist to predict, *a priori*, what will be the effect of a particular water on lead pipe under the conditions of ordinary practice. Next to no value attaches to experiments made by immersing strips of sheet lead in open or closed vessels containing the water under examination. In actual practice, many waters, which would be pronounced dangerous on the strength of such experiments, prove entirely harmless. The pipes very soon become covered with a naturally formed protective coating of difficultly soluble compounds of lead; and after a slight initial action, corrosion practically ceases if the pipes are kept constantly filled.

It may be said that while with most waters the action on the lead practically ceases, it probably never ceases absolutely. The water of Lake Cochituate, as supplied in Boston, Mass., through lead pipes, always contains traces of lead in solution. The amount of lead taken up by the water in passing through some 150 feet of pipe which had been in use for some years was found to be only 0.03 part in 100,000, or less than 0.02 grain in the U. S. gallon. Water which is allowed to remain in the pipe for some time, or is drawn from the hot-water faucets, may contain as much as 0.1, or even 0.2 part in 100,000 (from 0.06 to 0.12 grain in the gallon); and wherever lead distribution pipes are in use, it is safer always to run to waste enough water to clear the pipes, and never to use for drinking or for cooking water which has passed through the pipes while hot.

A similar precaution should be used in the case of new pipes; the water should be wasted intermittently but freely for a number of days. There is great difference in the susceptibility of different persons to lead poisoning. It is thought that as little as one fortieth of a grain to the gallon has caused sickness, but one tenth of a grain is usually regarded as an outside limit. It is doubtful whether there are any well-authenticated cases of lead poisoning from the use of the Cochituate water.

The Croton water supplied to New York City is similar to the Boston water in its action on lead, although at least one case of poisoning has been reported, which was supposed to be due to the daily use for some time of water which had stood over night in the pipes. The practical experience in the use of lead pipe in the cities mentioned, and in many others, shows that as a rule there is no danger in using lead pipes for house distribution in connection with a public supply.

The most unfavorable situation for lead pipe is as suction pipes in wells. Here the corrosion is often very rapid, and it is rendered more violent by the fact that the continual changes of level expose a longer or shorter portion of the pipe to the alternate action of air and water. There are instances enough of lead poisoning from this cause.

It may be remarked, in this connection, that the lead pipe now in use, at least in the eastern part of the country, is much inferior in strength and durability, and apparently more readily corroded, than that formerly in use. The lead now in the market has been desilverized by the zinc process, and this seems to give it a particular and disadvantageous character.

Other materials than lead are used in the house service. To block-tin or to tin-lined lead pipes, if the latter are properly made and properly put together, there is no objection on sanitary grounds. The corrosion of the tin by ordinary waters would result in the formation of insoluble and harmless substances. As to the suitability of the brass pipes which have been proposed, there seems to be no exact information. To the various sorts of "enamelled" wrought-iron pipes which are in the market there is no sanitary objection. The coating or enamel is generally some preparation of coal tar, with or without linseed oil, and this sort of pipe is particularly adapted for use in wells, where a portion of the outer surface is exposed alternately to the action of air and water; unfortunately, the coating is not always perfect, and when the original surface of the pipe is exposed, rusting begins. Zincked or "galvanized" iron, as it is called, is fully as bad in respect to rusting. The pipes are prepared by dipping the iron, previously well cleaned by means of dilute acid, into a bath of melted zinc. The zinc adheres firmly to the surface of the iron, and penetrates it to a certain extent, so that we do not deal with a simple coating such as we have on tinned iron, or on the various forms of enamelled pipe. The idea is that the zinc shall protect the iron by virtue of a galvanic action between the two metals, and it does protect the iron for a time. When the pipes are exposed to the action of water, corrosion begins at once : at first, the action is on the zinc alone, provided the original iron was free from rust, and the treatment with zinc was thorough ; but after a time the zinc which remains will cease to protect the iron, and iron-rust will begin to form. As regards this action, it is simply a question of time. Water that has passed through zincked pipes will be found almost always, if not invariably, to contain zinc compounds either in solution or in suspension ; the amount, however, is generally very small. As to the effect of such water on health there is some difference of opinion, but it is generally believed that the pipes may be safely used.

One of the best materials for service pipes is wrought-iron protected by the Bower-Barff process, provided practical experience justifies the theoretical expectations. To such pipes, coupled without the use of red or white lead, there can be nothing superior from a sanitary point of view, and for use in wells and cisterns they will supply a very serious want. Ordinary wrought-iron pipes, although possessing many advantages, have the great disadvantage of rusting very readily : the iron-rust is harmless but unsightly in drinking water, and may render the water unfit for culinary purposes and for use in the laundry.

Popular Tests.

The writer has little sympathy with popular tests. It is true that the observations on odor and taste and color may be made by a person who is not a chemist. There are also certain qualitative tests that any intelligent person can learn to make satisfactorily, and which would serve as indications to the chemist. It is in general true of popular tests, that they are apt to lead either to an unjustified sense of security or to an unnecessary feeling of alarm. The following test for sewage contamination, proposed by Heisch, and recommended by others, has some value.

Put some of the water (say half a pint) into a clean, colorless, glass-stoppered bottle, add a few grains of white sugar, shake until the sugar has dissolved, and leave the bottle freely exposed to the light in a warm room for a week or ten days. If the water becomes turbid, it is open to suspicion of sewage contamination; if it remains clear, it is probably safe.

Collection of Samples.

In connection with the chemical examination of water, the importance of taking due care in the collection of samples may be alluded to. The best vessel for collecting water for analysis is a glass-stoppered bottle; a clean demijohn which has never been used for any other purpose and which is stopped with a new and clean cork answers perfectly well, and is often more convenient. Tin cans or stoneware jugs are not suitable.

Considerable care is necessary in order to get a fair sample of the water. The demijohn should be rinsed several times thoroughly with the water to be collected and finally filled not quite to the mouth. The cork should be washed with the same water, and the demijohn stoppered tightly. The stopper should be tied over with a piece of cloth or "bandage gum," and the string sealed with sealing-wax, that the water may not be tampered with in transit.

If the water be taken from a pump or from a faucet, enough water should be pumped or allowed to run to waste to thoroughly clear the pipes. In taking water from a pond or river, it will generally be most convenient to use a clean crockery pitcher, which may be filled by plunging it beneath the surface (so as to avoid any scum or floating material), and then emptied into the demijohn; or a new and clean tin dipper may be employed. If a glass bottle is used, it may be plunged directly into the water and thus filled. In taking water from a river, the middle of the stream should be chosen if only one sample is taken.

TEA.

The tea plant, *Thea Sinensis*, an evergreen, and closely allied to the genus Camellia, is a native of China, Japan, and the north of Eastern India. The finest tea of China is grown between the twenty-seventh and thirty-first parallels of north latitude. But the plant will flourish from the equator to forty degrees north latitude.

Tea has been used as a beverage by the Chinese for ages past. Tradition refers to it as early as the third century. It first became known to Europeans about the end of the sixteenth century. Until the middle of the seventeenth, the price was from twenty-five to fifty dollars a pound; and a remarkable feature in its history is the reduction which has taken place in its commercial value, tea now being sold at Canton at from fifteen to twenty cents a pound, and in this country at fifty cents to one dollar. Tea is used at present by about one third of the human race. The consumption per head in Great Britain in 1835 was less than one and a half pounds. In 1877 it was four and a half pounds. In the United States in 1876 it was one and a half pounds. Among European nations tea is preeminently an English, Russian, and Dutch drink.

The quality of tea depends upon its flavor, which should be delicate and yet full; and this is affected by the time of gathering, whether or not the first of the four yearly gatherings, by the age of the tree, by the country in which it is grown, by the quality of the soil, and by the situation of the plantation. The two classes of tea, the black and the green, are produced in the same region, and often from the same trees. Green tea is rolled and dried very quickly, the whole process being finished in an hour or two, so that the leaf keeps its color. The idea that green tea is obtained by drying the leaves in copper pans is a popular error, which has been persisted in for a long time, without a shadow of truth for its foundation. For black tea the leaves are beaten and exposed to the air for some time, so that a sort of fermentation sets in. The production of the aromatic flavors is due to the processes of drying, since the leaves when freshly plucked have neither the odor nor flavor of the dried leaves. Hence different qualities of tea may be made from the same leaves, according to the treatment while drying. This is the source of the various kinds found in the market under the names Hyson, Oolong, etc. Some teas are scented with fragrant leaves.

Substitutes for tea are found in nearly every country. Sage leaves were frequently so used in England, a century ago. Labrador tea was prepared by the native American tribes. The leaves of thirty-two plants are known to have been thus used.

The important constituent of tea is an alkaloid called *theine*. It is present in varying proportions, from one to four per cent. The theine is supposed to be in combination with tannin, which is the most abundant soluble substance in tea, usually from sixteen to twenty-seven per cent. To the tannin is due the constipating effect of tea. The longer the tea leaves are steeped, the more tannin the solution contains. Regard for the lining of one's stomach would lead one to avoid all steeped teas. The infusion should be prepared immediately before drinking.

The odor and flavor of tea are due to an essential oil which is present in very small quantity, and which is developed during the roasting and drying. For a good tea, the volatile oil must not escape. To make a good pot of tea, scald out the pot with boiling hot soft water, place the tea in it as soon as possible, pour over it the boiling water, and close the pot immediately: allow it to stand in a hot place for a few minutes, but do not let it boil. Tea as drunk in China is always taken clear, without any addition of milk or sugar. The Russians add a few drops of lemon.

Lo-Yu, a learned Chinese who lived somewhere about 700 A. D., says of the effect of an infusion of tea, that it tempers the spirits and harmonizes the mind, dispels lassitude and relieves fatigue, awakens thought and prevents drowsiness, lightens or refreshes the body, and clears the perceptive faculties. Modern writers claim that tea excites the brain to increased activity, while it soothes and stills the vascular system, and hence its use in inflammatory diseases, and as a cure for headache. Taken in excess, it has the effect of a vegetable poison. It affects different people differently, and when it causes nervous excitement its use should be avoided. The infusion is stimulating and not nutritive; hence the use of tea and toast, so common among the workingwomen of America, is very poor economy, and is an evil, one had almost said, second only to the use of alcohol. Indeed, it has been called the tobacco of women; for while the tea does undoubtedly allow one to live on less food, it does not supply the place of food for any length of time. If the exhausted leaves were eaten after the infusion was drunk, as is the case in several countries, it would be more economical, since they contain about twenty per cent of nitrogenous matter, insoluble in water. On the coast of South America and on the slopes of the Himalayas the spent leaves are handed round among the company, sometimes on a silver salver, and much relished. In some places the leaves are powdered and mixed with various nutritious substances, and eaten without infusion.

According to the best authorities tea should not be drunk as a beverage by persons under middle age, as it is liable to interfere with the development of the nervous system. But for elderly and delicate people whose stomachs are incapable of digesting much food the use of tea is often valuable, as it, like coffee, prevents the waste of tissue, or, in other words, a person requires less food when tea is taken; but it should not be used for this purpose by working people, since it tells upon the digestive power of the stomach, and nothing can supply day after day the lack of nutritious food. Physicians now recognize a tea dyspepsia, and no one with a hope for better digestion should drink tea constantly three times a day.

Adulterations of Tea.

When tea was ten dollars a pound there was great temptation to mix other leaves with the genuine, or even to substitute them entirely; also to add to the weight by iron filings, etc., or sand gummed on plumbago and soapstone; the exhausted leaves were also used. Since the price has fallen, very much less adulteration is practised. It will not pay to work over the tea leaves to any extent, yet they are occasionally adulterated, and inferior grades due to carelessness in preparation and to less careful cultivation are quite common. In England all tea is sampled and inspected, and in 1879, of five hundred and seventy-five specimens examined, only three were found to require special disposal, — one damaged by water, one consisting of exhausted leaves, and one sanded.

The addition of mineral matter may be detected by burning a weighed quantity — one gram or more — in a platinum dish, and weighing the ash. Good tea gives from five to seven per cent of ash. If the leaves are exhausted, the per cent will be less. To ascertain the strength of the tea an infusion is the best test. If the decoction is very high-colored, the tea has probably been doctored. If there is not much extract, the leaves have been exhausted. The surest test of this is the specific gravity of the solution; but even this is a delicate test, since the specific gravity of a solution of two hundred grains of tea in two thousand grains of water is from 1.012 to 1.014, while that of exhausted leaves is 1.003 to 1.0057. Good tea should yield twenty-six per cent, and often as much as thirty-six per cent, of its weight to boiling water.

Dr. Farquharson of Iowa reports: "The proper examination of tea is a difficult and delicate task, only to be undertaken by an expert, who combines the attainments of a chemist, a microscopist, and a tea-taster." The most frequent coloring-matters or facings now in use are Prussian-blue and indigo. Prussian-blue may be detected by the addition of a solution of potash. This causes the color to disappear, but it can be restored by an acid. Indigo is not affected by potash in the cold, but is decomposed by permanganate of potash. The readiest method of detecting the addition of other kinds of leaves is by the microscope; but this of course requires training in the use of the instrument, and a knowledge of the appearance of the real tea leaves. The quantity of Prussian-blue mixed with gypsum or clay is about one grain to the ounce: probably not one third of this is Prussian-blue, so that the dose is homœopathic.

The Russians are said to have the most delicious tea of any nation in Europe. They have an inland trade with China, and choice teas are directly imported, without exposure to the heat and close air of the hold of a vessel, so injurious to teas of a delicate flavor. Their method of making tea also has much to do with its fine flavor, and as samovars are a national feature, and now beginning to be imported and used in this country, I will endeavor to describe them and their use.

The samovar is a large brass urn, lined with block tin. The urn and the stand which raises it from the table are all in one piece, in those I have seen. The urns hold from four to eight quarts of water, which is poured in through a small hole, three quarters of an inch in diameter, in the top, and they are emptied by a stop-cock or faucet, like any hot-water urn. The fire for heating the water is arranged in this way. Directly through the centre of the urn, from top to bottom, runs a hollow cylinder, which is closed below by a little grate, the bars of which show below the body of the urn. These bars are fine enough to prevent any fire from falling upon the tray or table on which it stands, and the urn stands sufficiently high from the table to prevent any danger from heat. The metal of the stand is solid below, so there is no danger from fire. At the upper end the cylinder rises above the urn an inch or two, and has a tall chimney of brass, that can be taken off by its odd straight handle, as required.

It is usually one servant's duty in Russia to take care of the samovar, to fill it with the freshest of water, to kindle the fire, and to bring it in when all is ready for the table. A twist of paper is placed in the bottom of the cylinder, with some splinters of kindling wood.

Upon this are placed bits of charcoal broken into bits the size of walnuts. The Russians themselves often have a special charcoal made from cocoa-nuts, the hard shells making a very dense, odorless charcoal, which gives off an intense heat. The fire is lighted from the grate below. The chimney is put on, and the fire is allowed to burn until all smoke and smell from the wood and paper have passed away, and the charcoal is in a glow. Then it is carried in and set upon the table.

As soon as the water sends out a jet of steam from the hole at the top, beside the cylinder, the tea is made by the hostess. Now notice that the water has just reached the boiling point. It has lost none of its life or air. It is simply fresh, pure water brought to the boiling point. The teapot is made scalding hot, and the tea is taken from a caddy upon the table. At first only a little water is poured upon it. The chimney is taken off and the tea-pot is set upon the cylinder over the glowing coals, upon the same principle as setting the tea-pot in the top of the boiling tea-kettle on the fire, as we often see done here in our kitchens. In a few moments, more boiling water is added, and the tea-pot replaced over the coals. The tea is poured into the cups when it has steeped sufficiently long, sugar is added, and instead of cream a slice of lemon is slipped into each cup. Fresh tea and water are put in the tea-pot, and it is again placed over the coals.

To empty the water from the samovar, it is sufficient to let it run out from the faucet. This is first done, and then the coal and ashes are shaken out by turning the samovar upside down, as it does not take apart. But in Russia the samovar is often kept hot the greater part of the day, fresh charcoal and water being occasionally added as required, until the time comes for a fresh samovar to be made ready for the table.

COFFEE.

One tradition relates that, in antique days, a poor dervish, who lived in a valley of Arabia Felix, observed a strange hilarity in his goats on their return home every evening. To find out the cause of this, he watched them closely one day, and observed that they eagerly devoured the blossoms and fruit of a tree he had hitherto disregarded. He tried the effect of this food upon himself, and was thrown into such a state of exhilaration that his neighbors accused him of having drunk of the forbidden wine; but he revealed to them his discovery, and they at once agreed that Allah had sent the coffee plant to the faithful as a substitute for the wine.

The name of coffee is given to a beverage prepared from the seeds of plants, which are roasted, ground, and infused in boiling water. The seeds most used are those of the Arabian coffee tree (an evergreen, *Caffea Arabica*), which belongs to the natural order Cinchonaceæ, the same order to which belongs the tree from which is obtained the Peruvian bark of commerce. It is probable that the use of coffee has been known from time immemorial in Abyssinia, where the tree is native. In Persia it is known to have been in use as early as A. D. 875.

The first allusion to coffee in an English book is believed to be in Burton's Anatomy of Melancholy: "The Turks have a drink called coffee, (for they use no wine,) so named of a berry as black as soot, and as bitter, which they sup up as warm as they can suffer, because they find by experience that that kind of drink, so used, helpeth digestion and produceth alacrity."

While in Mahometan countries its use as an antisoporific in the long devotional exercises rendered it obnoxious to the conservative priests, — and while some held it to be an intoxicant, and so prohibited by the Koran, in England it seems to have been opposed by liquor-dealers, who alleged that the popularity of the coffee-houses was so great as to draw away their custom. The popularity of the coffee-houses also aroused suspicion of disloyalty in the gatherings, so that they were made the object of a royal proclamation by Charles II. in 1675.

Coffee was introduced into England about the same time as tea, and its use increased very rapidly, until it reached its maximum in 1854, when the import into Great Britain was 37,441,373 pounds. Since then the consumption has decreased, partly owing to a greater use of tea, and partly to the increase of coffee substitutes. The amount per head used in Great Britain was one and a quarter pounds in 1857; in 1875-77, only three fourths of a pound. In the United States it is about eight pounds; in Holland and Germany, about fourteen.

The introduction of coffee into Europe was bitterly opposed, and the use of it denounced from the pulpit.

Nevertheless the tree has been cultivated in all tropical countries which have been colonized by Europeans. Brazil now supplies two thirds of the coffee of the world.

The most valuable constituent of coffee is *caffeine*, an alkaloid identical with the theine of tea. There is present about one per cent of it. The peculiar flavor and aroma of coffee are due to one or more oils or fats, which become changed to peculiar aromatic compounds in the roasting. There are some thirteen per cent of these, and they probably possess the stimulating properties noticed in the infusion. Caffeic acid, an astringent somewhat like the tannin of tea, is present, but only from three to five per cent. Hence, the action of coffee is not as deleterious to the coatings of the stomach as is that of tea. Coffee also contains sugar to five or seven per cent, which is all converted into caramel in roasting.

The exhausted berries also contain nutritious nitrogenous matter, and some Eastern nations drink grounds and all. In Sumatra the leaves are used, and seem to have a large proportion of the properties of the berry.[1]

---

[1] See Chemistry of Common Life, p. 141.

The effect of coffee on the human system is to counteract the tendency to sleep, and it is almost certain that it was this property which originally led to its use as a beverage. It also excites the nervous system, and when taken in excess produces contractions and tremors of the muscles, and a feeling of buoyancy and exhilaration somewhat similar to that produced by alcohol, but does not end with depression or collapse. Professor Johnstone thus describes the properties and effects of coffee: "It exhilarates, arouses, and keeps awake; it counteracts the stupor occasioned by fatigue, by disease, or opium; it allays hunger to a certain extent; it gives to the weary increased strength and vigor, and imparts a feeling of comfort and repose." Its physiological effects upon the system, so far as they have been investigated, appear to be, that, while it makes the brain more active, it soothes the body generally, makes the change and waste of matter slower, and the demand for food in consequence less.

For soldiers and travellers exposed to great hardships, coffee is the best agent known for restoration of the exhausted energies. Its use can be abused, like that of any other good thing, but, used understandingly, coffee is an important addition to one's diet.

The adulterations of coffee are mostly seeds, as beans or pease; or roots, as chiccory, dandelion, and carrots. As yet, there has been no seed found which, when roasted and ground, corresponds with coffee, either in its physiological properties or in the chemical composition.

The detection of the presence of chiccory, caramel, and some of the sweet roots, as turnips, carrots, and parsnips, is quite easy. If a few grains of the suspected sample are placed on the surface of water in a glass vessel, beaker, or tumbler, each particle of chiccory, etc., will become surrounded by a yellow-brown cloud, which rapidly diffuses through the water until the whole becomes colored.

Pure coffee, under the same conditions, gives no sensible color to the water until after the lapse of about fifteen minutes. Caramel (burnt sugar) of course colors the water very deeply. Dandelion-root gives a deeper color than coffee, but not as deep as chiccory; the same is true of bread raspings. Both these adulterations may be more readily detected by the taste, and the bread by its softening. Beans and pease give much less color to the water than pure coffee; they can be readily detected by the microscope, as can roasted figs and dates, or date-stones. But as was said under tea, the microscopical examination must be made by one who has skill. The use of the microscope is not to be learned in one lesson. In months of practice one sees more and more each time the instrument is used, so that, while it is an invaluable aid to those accustomed to its use, it is as unreliable as the chemical tests in the hands of the unskilled.[1]

The preparation of good coffee requires only an understanding of its properties, and is not as difficult or as dependent upon complicated apparatus as is often supposed. Raw coffee, when kept dry, improves with age. The best Java is said to be some seven or eight years old. To prepare the kernel for use, it must first be properly roasted by a quick heat, like that used for popping corn. The kernels should swell and pop in much the same way, though not to the same extent. When the flavor has thus been developed, and the berry made brittle, it is to be ground in a mill or pounded in a mortar as fine as may be, and then, to obtain the full strength, placed in an earthen-ware vessel, covered with cold water, allowed to stand for

---

[1] For illustrations of the appearance of tea leaves, and other leaves and berries, see Bell, Hassall, Blyth, and König.

some hours, and brought to the boiling heat just before use. While this is the most economical treatment, most people prepare an infusion made by pouring boiling water upon the fine coffee. The vessel should then be closed and allowed to stand at a boiling heat for five to ten minutes: it should never boil violently, as the delicate aroma of the coffee is then lost. "Coffee, to be good, must be made strong. From one to two ounces to a pint of water is recommended; three times the volume of milk may then be added. This is better than to add water. In countries where the best coffee is made, there is a concurrence of opinion that roasted coffee should not come in contact with any metal; but that it should be powdered in a wooden mortar, kept in glass or porcelain, and infused in porcelain or earthen-ware jugs, or other closed vessels." An expensive method of preparation is by the percolation of boiling water through the coffee, drop by drop. The simplest apparatus for this is a flannel bag suspended in the coffee-pot, and which carries the coffee.

COCOA.

The cocoa of commerce is chiefly prepared from the seeds of the plant *Theobroma cacao,* which grows in the West Indies, Brazil, and Guiana; also in some parts of Asia and Africa.

The term *theobroma* implies food for the gods, and the name was given to the plant by Linnæus, who is said to have been very fond of the beverage prepared from cocoa. The Mexicans called it *cacaoa quahuitl,* and the beverage *chocolatl;* and we probably derive from these native names our words *cocoa* and *chocolate.* It was introduced into Europe by the Spaniards in 1520, and appears to have been known to the inhabitants of Central America from time immemorial. England uses about five ounces per head annually.

The cocoa bean contains fifty per cent of fat, thirteen per cent of nitrogenous substance, half of which is soluble, about seven per cent of a tannin-like principle, four per cent of starch, and about one per cent of theobromine, an alkaloid resembling theine. Thus it combines in a remarkable way the important substances which constitute a perfect food, and it is not strange that it holds so high a place in popular favor, yet the large percentage of fat renders it too rich to be taken as an addition to an otherwise hearty meal: hence the various preparations in which the most of the fat is extracted. A cup of cocoa taken with milk is in itself a nutritive drink, — almost of the nature of soup, since cocoa is not soluble, only held in suspension.

Cocoa nibs are the cracked beans; but since some time is required to soften them, the prepared forms are preferred, with or without the fat, *chocolate* having more fat than some other preparations. *Shells* are the husks destitute of the fat, but containing more astringent substance.

The chief additions to chocolate and prepared cocoa are starch and sugar. Sometimes ferruginous earths have been found, and occasionally foreign fats are used.

In making tea we make an infusion. In making coffee we make either an infusion or a decoction. Now in making cocoa from the nibs or the cracked cocoa, we make a decoction; that is, the cocoa must actually boil. If it stands upon the stove or range, and steeps without boiling, we have an infusion, and we obtain as a result an intensely bitter drink. But if it boils, — and it is an important, curious fact the difference a few degrees of heat will make, — we have a smooth, oily, nutty beverage, which is most agreeable to drink, and very nutritious also, which the bitter beverage is not. There is the same difference between an infusion and a decoction of coffee, but the bitter of coffee is not so unpleasant nor so marked. Tea, on the contrary, and also all herb teas, like mint, catnip, etc., are harsh and bitter when boiled, losing all their fragrance and delicate flavor. Tea is more of a mere beverage than coffee, which approaches a liquid food, though not as nearly as cocoa does.

III.

CEREAL FOODS. — BARLEY, RICE, OATS, MAIZE, RYE, AND WHEAT.

THE cereals all belong to the family of grasses, and some member of the group flourishes in every latitude. Barley grows even within the Arctic Circle, and thence southward are found, in the following order, oats, rye, wheat, maize, while within the tropics rice is found. The seeds of these plants have been used for the food of man from time immemorial. The Egyptians have a tradition that barley was the first to be so used. They are the most important of all food substances.

A general description will serve for all the seeds or kernels. The shape is from round to oval or oblong, with a groove on one side running the length of the kernel. This indentation serves to protect the germ which it encloses. Outside the germ are usually recognized three layers. The outer layer, which serves to hold the inner ones compactly together and to keep them dry, is made up chiefly of woody fibre, or cellulose, and is comparatively worthless for the purpose of nutrition. Next, there are in most grains one or more layers of cells which contain nitrogenous and phosphatic compounds, while within, forming the body of the seed, is found the mass of starch granules, larger and smaller, with intermingled cells of the glutinous or albuminoid constituents. All these are supported in a loose framework of cellular tissue. The proportion of these constituents varies greatly in the different grains and in varieties of the same grain. Rice has the largest proportion of starch, and oats contain the most oily and phosphatic material.

The term *flour* is often used to designate the meal or powder obtained by the grinding of any species of grain or seed. But the use of the word in the United States is for the most part limited to the finely ground portion, the more starchy portion; while by the term *meal* — a Saxon word meaning finely ground, soft to the touch — is understood the bran or the product of the grinding of the whole grain. Both terms are generic, and are qualified by a descriptive adjective; as, wheat flour, corn meal, etc.

Barley and rice are for the most part cooked whole,

oats and maize are coarsely crushed, while wheat and rye are finely ground and separated into the flour or white sifted starch and gluten, and the husk or bran which is left after the bolting, as the sifting is technically called.

BARLEY.

Barley belongs to the genus Hordeum. It is probably a native of Northern or Central Asia, but it has a remarkable power of adapting itself to a great range of temperature, and has a wider distribution than wheat or oats. On the Eastern continent its culture extends from 70° north latitude to 42° south, and in America from 62° north to 20° south. Its use as an article of food is coeval with the history of man. It yields a greater produce per acre than any other grain except rice. It was largely cultivated by the Romans, and used chiefly as food for horses. In England, in the middle of the seventeenth century, it was commonly used as the food of the people, because it grew readily in any part of the kingdom. Since improved means of transportation have brought all countries within a few days of each other, wheat is carried to lands in which it will not thrive, and people no longer need to live on the produce of their own soil. Barley has less starch, and more cellulose, mineral matter, and fat, than rice. It is at present largely used for the manufacture of beer, being better suited for it than the other grains.

RICE.

The rice of commerce is the product of the grass *Oryza sativa*, probably a native of the East Indies, but cultivated in all portions of tropical and sub-tropical regions. It forms the principal food of nearly one third of the human race, and enters largely into the diet of all civilized nations; although, on account of the excess of starch over the nitrogenous and mineral constituents, it has been said that rice can only be the substantive article of diet of an indolent and feeble people. The outer coat of woody fibre does not adhere closely, and is easily removed, so that, as sent to market, the shelled grain is the inner or starch kernel. The wild rice of North America belongs to another genus, *Zinania aquatica*. It grows in the north temperate regions, and deserves more notice than it has hitherto received. Rice flour is now largely used in the adulteration of many finely ground foods and of condiments.

OATS.

Oatmeal is prepared from two species, *Avena sativa* and *Avena orientalis*, which belong to the same natural order as wheat. This grain grows best in a cool, moist climate. The native country of the grass is not known with certainty. There is evidence that the plant was known in Britain in 1296, and mention is made of the use of oatmeal porridge as an article of food in 1596. In 1698 the consumption of oatmeal was second only to barley, but wheat has gradually taken its place in Southern England. By kiln-drying and removing the husk, groats or grits are obtained, which, when ground, yield oatmeal. The husk is not as completely removed as in the case of rice, and the meal is not as white as wheat meal. Although it contains a large proportion of nitrogenous matter it is not in the form of the tenacious gluten of wheat: hence it will not make light or porous bread. Oatmeal is not as easily digested as wheat flour, and as a staple article of diet it is best suited to persons who are much in the open air; but a portion of the morning meal may advantageously be of this very nutritious grain. Blyth says that in England it is sometimes adulterated with barley meal.

MAIZE.

Maize, *Zea mays*, is remarkable in the order of grasses for the large size of its grains, and for the heads into which they are collected. It grows wild in the neighborhood of Mexico and in tropical America, and has now been introduced into every quarter of the globe, though it cannot be relied upon as a field crop in Great Britain. It has been said, that what wheat is in Europe and rice in Asia, maize is in America.

Maize, or Indian corn as it is called in the United States, was not much consumed in England until the year of the potato famine, in 1846, when hominy was imported. Now about 8,000,000 pounds are annually imported, chiefly from the Black and Mediterranean Sea borders. It is an excellent food, easily digested, and very nutritious. It is much used for the preparation of starch and for "infant's foods." The starch is separated, and used in place of the more costly arrowroot.

MILLET.

Millet, *Panicum miliaceum*, also a native of tropical countries, is one of the largest fodder grasses, often called Guinea grass or Guinea corn. This grain is used for human food only in hot countries. It is very nutritious, and, so far as composition shows, is quite equal to wheat.

RYE.

Rye, *Secale cerale*, is nearly allied to wheat. The grains are smaller, and the flour not so white. It is very rich in nitrogenous substances. It grows a little farther north than wheat flourishes, and it thrives on a sandy soil, too poor for any other grain. The bread made from rye flour is not so white and light as that made from wheat flour, but it is extensively used in Europe. The chief objection to its use is, that it is liable to be injured by a fungus, which produces an appearance like a spur, and which is called *ergot*. If these swelled grains are ground with the others, the flour is rendered unwholesome, and even dangerous.

WHEAT.

Wheat flour is prepared from the seeds of the genus Triticum. The two varieties commonly cultivated are *Triticum hybernum*, and the bearded wheat, *Triticum æstivum*. The cultivation of wheat has superseded that of all other grains in climates where it will thrive, (in the temperate zone as far as 60° north,) but in the Middle Ages it was food only for the wealthy classes. Its use has been constantly on the increase, until it is now food for all classes.

The reason seems to be, that bread made from it has no unpleasant or pronounced taste, so that the most fastidious palate does not become weary of it, and has a light, spongy or porous character, quite peculiar to the wheat loaf. This adapts it for ready digestion, and is due to the peculiar nature of gluten, which in good flour is very elastic, and, when the moistened dough is compressed, causes it to spring back again to its place.

The quality of the prepared flour is dependent upon the variety of wheat, the curing of the ripened grain, and the process of grinding.

There are two kinds of wheat, the hard and the soft, which are referred to in the description of the grinding.

The curing of wheat is of the utmost importance, for if the grain is allowed to become damp and mouldy, a disagreeable flavor will be communicated to the flour.

For grinding, two processes are used, which are known as high and low milling. In early times the kernels were brayed in a mortar, and later they were ground between stones. Low milling is a grinding between two large, round stones, one or both revolving at so small a distance from each other as to crush the kernels, which are caught, as it were, by radial grooves in the stones. The wheat is often moistened in grinding, as it is thought to be more readily crushed. The heat developed is considerable, so that the temperature of the flour as it comes from the stones is about 120° F. The heating, and the grinding of a portion of the husk so fine that it sifts with the body of the grain, are the chief objections to this method. The action is purely a single crushing, and is better adapted for the softer kinds of wheat than high milling, which is a succession of crackings, or of slight and partial crushings, alternating with sifting and sorting.

For this process the hard wheats, such as the Hungarian, are adapted. In general, the method may be described as follows. A series of cylindrical rolls is arranged at distances so graded that, when the wheat kernel passes between the first set, it is merely cracked; then the fragments drop between the next set, and are again cracked; and so on. In this way the husk is not bruised, only flattened out and loosened, so that the dry starch granules drop out. The flour is not heated, since it is not subjected to friction, and since it falls through the cool air between each set of rolls. It is thought that the separation of the non-nutritious portion is also more complete, and hence that the flour is richer in the phosphates and nitrogenous substances, which are found in the layer of cells next the husk. Since there are no particles of bran in the high-milled flour, it is whiter, and since it has been ground dry, it has less moisture and will keep longer.

It is thought that the heat developed in low milling may change somewhat the character of the gluten, rendering it less tenacious, and so the flour less fit for the making of light bread. Doubtless this has its influence, since it is well known that the same brand of flour will differ at different times, without any apparent reason.

There is also a mixture of the two processes called half high milling. A plan has also been tried, with some success, of pulverizing the grains by friction of the kernels upon each other, the wheat being kept in motion by beaters revolving at a high velocity in a hollow cylinder.

The next step in the production of flour is the sifting and sorting. The sifting is generally done by a series of sieves, and finally by bolt cloth, — a fine silk cloth. This gives the fine flour, while the coarser grades are left by the way.

Low milling yields about eighty per cent of flours of various grades, differing comparatively little from each other. High milling, on the other hand, yields only about forty-five per cent of the choicest flour, such as the famous Vienna bread is made from, with several inferior grades.

Flour for household use will perhaps average seventy per cent of starch and dextrine, about seven per cent each of sugar, mineral matter, and cellulose, one per cent of fat, and about fifteen per cent of albuminous or nitrogenous substances. These constituents are so proportioned as to render wheat flour a highly nutritious food, capable by itself of sustaining life and health.

The following account of a visit to one of the large flour mills in Minnesota, in 1884, will be of interest : —

"The wheat is poured into the mill from the elevator, and sent up from the basement to the upper or seventh story by steam power, the mill being seven stories high.

"The first process is sorting and cleaning the wheat. Any bits of iron, nails, straw, or bits of wood, are thrown out as it passes through the cleansing-machines. Seeds of weeds, such as cockle (*Lychnis Githago*), grass seeds, and the shrivelled grains of the wheat itself, are all separated or sifted out. The wheat is passed between brush rollers, and all dust removed, so that a handful of grain examined in this stage shows plump, even-sized kernels, which seem almost polished, so beautifully clean are they.

"In the next process, the grain is cracked once longitudinally, that is, in a line with the groove; it is then crushed again, and then a third time. This third time the husk lies free from the grain, and is a mere film of tissue.

"The method of cracking the grain is comparatively new, and is thought to take all the wheat, and leave nothing in the husk as a rule. Here and there a husk could be picked out with an atom adherent, but rarely.

"The wheat is now bolted through coarse sieves,

which take out this husk or bran, and leave the wheat like a meal, called 'Middlings.' This is very sweet when chewed a moment. The bran is run down into cars and sold for feeding stock, and the demand is always greater than the supply.

"The middlings are now ground and bolted five times, looking very much like flour the last time. This flour is now bolted through fine silk sieves, which are cylinders revolving on a horizontal axis. On opening the boxes to look in on these sieves, there comes out a warm, sweet smell, with an odor like that of new bread.

"*Summary of Processes.*

"First of all, the grain is cleaned and sorted.
1. The grain cracked lengthwise.
2. The grain crushed.
3. Husk now loose, with the kernel crushed.
4. Bolted. The result, Bran, and No. 1 Middlings.
5. Middlings No. 2.
6. Middlings No. 3, finer still.
7. Middlings No. 4, finer still.
8. Middlings No. 5, finer still.
9. Middlings are now like flour.
10. This flour is ground once more and bolted.

"To be packed, the flour comes down large cylinders into barrels or bags. The packing is all automatic, only one man being required at a machine. But there are a number of machines in operation in a row, on each side of the mill.

"When filled, the barrel or bag is slipped upon the scales and weighed, the workman adding or taking away flour, so as to make the weight (196 lbs. to a barrel) exact. Flour for shipping abroad is usually put into sacks or bags of various sizes, as it is more easily handled and better stowed in this form.

"The flour from summer wheat is considered the best for bread, but it requires more kneading.

"Every improvement is added to insure safety in the mill, to lighten the labor, and to increase the amount and quality of the flour produced. Attached to the machinery are tubes, which, by an exhaust, draw away all the impalpable dust from around the cylinders, and also take it from the air of the room. This fine dust becomes inflammable when it is electrical, and it becomes electrical in contact with the revolving machinery. The great explosion at one of the Washburn mills is presumed to have been due to this cause, and the spark which touched it off a bit of fine iron wire in the wheat, which became red-hot passing through the rollers. This is one reason also for the extreme care used in cleaning the wheat before grinding, lest any bit of iron should pass through the machinery.

"The dust drawn from the air, with the sweepings from the boxes and shafts, is saved and used in the inferior grades of flour."

The adulteration of flour is probably not practised to any great extent in this land of cheap wheat. In books relating to the food of foreign countries, reference is always made to the admixture of the inferior sorts of grain, to mineral additions for increasing the weight, such as chalk or gypsum, and to the addition of alum or copper sulphate, in order to enable the baker to make whiter bread out of an inferior grade of flour. It is said that the gluten becomes softer and less elastic and tenacious when the flour has been over-heated in grinding, or if the heap of grain has been heated or fermented before grinding, and the like. It is found that a little alum added to the flour seems to restore the tenacity of the gluten, and render the flour capable of making better and whiter bread.

Microscopic examination will serve to detect the

first class of adulteration, the amount of ash (which should not exceed one per cent) will indicate the second, and a careful chemical analysis will show the third. It must be remembered, however, that the husk of the kernel contains some alumina, so that a trace may always be found in the ash. If the flour contains any considerable quantity of alum, it will turn blue when moistened with a solution of logwood.

The proportion of gluten is of great importance, if the flour is to make up a large portion of the diet of a family. The following method of determining it is given by Dietzsch (p. 173). A portion of flour weighing one hundred grams is made up to a stiff paste with forty to fifty grams of water, allowed to stand half an hour, placed in a cloth, and kneaded under a stream of running water until the water no longer comes through milky. The yellowish elastic residue should weigh, when moist, from thirty to thirty-five grams; when dry, fifteen to eighteen grams. If the paste stands three hours instead of half an hour, the residue is said to be some three per cent more.

The testing of flour in the barrel is, like tea-tasting, an acquired art. Only long practice can enable one to judge with certainty of the quality of flour by its shade of yellow, or its mode of caking when pressed, etc. The importance of good flour can hardly be over-estimated, since upon good bread depends the health of the greater part of the human race in all temperate climates.

BUCKWHEAT.

Buckwheat does not belong to the grasses or cereals, but to the family Polygonaceæ, which includes rhubarb and dock. It grows as far north as 72°, and thus stands next to barley. It matures very quickly, — in one hundred days, — and thrives on sandy soil. It is probably a native of Western Asia, and is largely grown in temperate countries. The seed, when stripped of its indigestible husk, which composes about twenty per cent of it, is rich in food material.

STARCHES, ETC.

The prepared starches are purified, so that they contain little else than pure starch, and thus are not capable of sustaining life by themselves. Starch may be derived from the cereal grains mentioned above, or from tubers or roots, as the potato, arrowroot, and manihot or yucca, which yields farina and tapioca, and from the stems of plants, as the sago palm.

Corn starch is much used in the United States as an article of diet. *Farina* is another name for a preparation from the starch of maize or wheat, which now takes the place of the farina of manihot.

Genuine *macaroni* and *vermicelli* are made from wheat rich in gluten, and hence are exceedingly nutritious. Imitations are made from flour colored with saffron, or other yellow coloring-matter.

Arrowroot is derived from plants of the genus Maranta, of the West India Islands and tropical America, the chief species being *M. arundinacea*. The earliest recorded notice of the plant, the knowledge of which was obtained from South American Indians, refers to the supposed virtue possessed by its roots as an antidote to poisoned arrows; and it probably derives its name from this. Arrowroot was introduced into England about the beginning of this century; but its use has been largely superseded by that of corn starch.

IV.

MILK, BUTTER, CHEESE.

MILK.

THE milk of animals has been used as human food from time immemorial. In early ages it was the milk of goats, asses, etc., which was common; now however, cow's milk is used all over the world.

Milk is often called the perfect food, since it contains all the elements necessary for nutrition, and in the right proportions. One of the greatest advances in modern medicine, as well as in wholesome living, is the recognition of milk as an article of diet, especially for invalids, young people, and fever patients. Most persons can digest it when a little lime water is added, if it does not suit them without it. It is essential, however, that the milk supplied be of good quality, and from healthy, well-fed animals.

Public attention is now being called to the quality of milk purchased, and it is to be hoped that vigilance will not be relaxed, although the question of the purity of milk is one of the most difficult with which the analyst has to deal, since genuine milk varies widely in composition, owing to the breed of the cows and the feeding and care which they receive. The two determinations upon which chemists chiefly rely are the percentage of fats (butter) and of the solids not fats. But the range of these in pure milk is wide; late investigations give the maximum and minimum as follows. Solids not fats, from 11.27 per cent down to 8 per cent; so that the analyst must require, as a rule, over 8.5 per cent. For the butter fats the highest amount given is 6.87 per cent, the lowest 1.92 per cent, but the requirement for good milk cannot well go above 2.4 per cent. Accurate analysis demands so much skill and practice that expert chemists only are, as a rule, competent to give an opinion on the quality of milk. The various instruments proposed, such as lactometers and lactoscopes, cannot be relied upon, especially in inexperienced hands.

The most frequent adulteration is water; coloring-matters are then added to give the requisite yellowness. Greater danger to health comes from the use of milk from diseased or improperly fed cows, than from any substances added to the milk, unless the water used is taken from a foul well. The fact that milk is so largely used by children and people in delicate health renders it indispensable that the quality of the milk should be of the very best. The moral sense of the community should demand this. Milk is very liable to undergo the so-called lactic fermentation, in which the sugar is changed to lactic acid; hence, the greatest precautions should be taken as to cleanliness of the vessels into which the liquid is poured.

The composition of milk may be roughly stated as follows: water, 86 per cent; lactose, or milk sugar, 5.5 per cent; milk fat, 4 per cent; caseine, or curd, 4 per cent; saline matter, 5 per cent. The fat is held in suspension in the liquid in the form of globules, of which it is estimated that there are about three and a half millions in every cubic millimeter.

CONDENSED MILK.

The extremely unstable character of milk, and the consequent difficulty of transportation and preservation for any length of time, have led to the adoption of various processes for concentrating the valuable constituents, which are only about fourteen per cent of the weight, into a smaller bulk and more stable condition. The usual process consists in simple concentration. The milk is evaporated in vacuum pans, and toward the end heated to 180° F., in order to destroy any germs of mould. It is put up in tin cans, sealed hermetically, and may then be kept any length of time. Sometimes a little sugar is added. In either case, the product is sold as condensed milk, which often contains about one third as much water as the original liquid.

CREAM.

When milk is allowed to stand at rest for some hours, the fat globules rise to the top, forming a layer from one tenth to one fifth of the total thickness. This layer, rich in fat, is called cream, and contains from twenty to forty per cent of fat.

BUTTER.

When cream or milk is agitated for some time (churned), the fat globules are collected into a more or less compact mass, called butter.

Butter is a very important article of diet, especially in English-speaking countries. It is of all animal fats the favorite, not only on account of its pleasant taste, but because it is the most easily digested.

Herodotus, in his account of the Scythians, makes an obscure mention of butter, and this is the earliest reference known. Dioscorides is the first to observe that, when melted and poured over vegetables, it serves the same purpose as oil, and that it can be used in pastry. It is not mentioned by Galen, or other writers of his time, as food, and indeed to this day it is little used in Southern countries, so that it might almost be said to be a product of Northern civilization in its present uses. There is undoubted evidence that butter was well known to the Anglo-Saxons, and used for salves and medicines.

Butter is prepared by separating the fats from the water and curd of milk by agitation, which causes the lighter particles of fat to rise to the top, which then are collected and worked into a homogeneous mass. This process seems to be very successfully accomplished at present by the centrifugal machine.

Good butter consists of fats, water, and curd. The water varies from eight to sixteen per cent. Over sixteen per cent is injurious to the keeping of butter. There should not be over one per cent of curd left, because it tends to grow rancid and mould, thus tainting the butter.

Butter is very sensitive to unpleasant odors, and must be kept with great care, in closed vessels, even a few hours' exposure to ordinary air injuring the delicate flavor. It would be well if all girls could serve an apprenticeship in a good dairy for a few weeks, in order to learn cleanliness. Most of the best butter is now made in large dairies or factories, where, owing to the amount of property at stake, the most scrupulous cleanliness is enforced.

The seventy-eight to ninety per cent of butter fats are for the most part identical with those in olive and palm oils, and in other animal fats; but the peculiar flavor of butter is due to the presence of five to eight per cent of butyric, capronic, caprylic, and caprinic acids. These fatty acids are much less stable than oleic, palmitic, and stearic acids, which are often called the fixed fatty acids. In butter, human fat, and goose fat, palmitic acid is the most abundant. It is so named from its occurrence in palm oil. Oleic acid is common to these fats, and to beef, mutton, and hog fats.

Stearic acid is found in small quantities in butter, while it is a chief and constant constituent of beef tallow.

During the Franco-German war, in 1870-71, a French chemist, Mége-Mouries, invented a process for obtaining from other animal fats the fatty acids common to them and to butter, and making from them a very fair artificial butter, for the use of the French army. The process has been further perfected by working the product with milk, sometimes with the addition of a little of the coloring-matter of butter and of a little butyric ether, so that neither in consistency nor in flavor is the artificial to be clearly distinguished from the real butter. This product, if well made, will keep longer than butter, and for many uses, such as cooking, is a valuable addition to the food materials of the world; but unfortunately it is not always sold under its own name, partly because the public is slow to accept a new article. People justly complain when they get oleomargarine instead of the more valuable butter which they pay for. It is a fraud upon their pockets, though not injurious to health.

There is probably no serious cause for alarm as to the quality of the fats used in making artificial butter, for the financial success of a large manufactory will be secured only by the good quality of the product. The name oleomargarine is derived from the fatty acids present, — oleic and margaric, as the mixture of stearic and palmitic acids was formerly called. Rarely has there been a fraud so difficult to detect, since not only the apparent but the real differences between genuine and artificial butter are but slight. Yet careful chemical analysis will show about eighty-seven per cent of fixed fatty acids in butter, and about ninety-five per cent in the fats used in making artificial butter.

Reichert's process of determining the volatile acids peculiar to butter answers well in skilled hands. An analytical chemist has little difficulty in deciding upon the quality of a suspected sample. The expense attending such an examination, however, prevents its application as often as is desirable. The detection of the crystals of the different fats, as proposed by Taylor, may be an important aid. Some simple and easily applied test is much to be desired, but the public yet waits its discovery.

CHEESE.

Good cheese is composed of the total solids of milk curdled by rennet before the milk sours. Poor cheese is made from skimmed milk and hence has less fat. Cheese is really a condensed milk, and is a valuable article of diet, replacing meat to a great extent with those whose stomachs it suits. One pound of cheese is estimated to contain as much nitrogenous substance as a pound or a pound and a half of beef. It has been very free from adulteration, but now oleomargarine and lard cheeses are reported as coming into market. The rind of the cheese may be brushed over with some metallic salt to preserve it from the attacks of fungi, etc., so that it is well to pare it off before eating.

CREAM CHEESE.

Cream cheese has come into favor and is now found in all groceries and milk depots. It is for most persons a wholesome and appetizing food, and is not liable to serious adulteration so far as is known to the writer.

"Filled cheese" is on the market quite openly in some quarters; that is, cheese made from skimmed milk from which the butter fat has been abstracted and other and cheaper fat substituted. This is, doubtless, somewhat less digestible than the whole-milk cheese, but its food value is otherwise quite as good.

The ripening of cheese by bacteria is discussed in Bulletin No. 25 from the office of Ex. Stations, U. S. Dept. of Agri., and in "The Story of Germ Life," by Prof. H. W. Conn.

V.

SUGAR.

THE word *sugar*, probably of Sanscrit origin, is now used to designate a class of substances possessing a sweet taste, and capable of breaking up into alcohol and carbon dioxide under the influence of ferments, such as yeast.

Of the various kinds of sugar known to chemists, only two or three are of importance in domestic economy; namely, cane sugar, and grape sugar, or *glucose*, as it is often called.

Common sugar is called cane sugar, because it is obtained principally from the sugar cane, a tall grass, *Saccharum officinarum*, a native of Southern Asia. It is the sweetest of all the sugars, and is technically called *sucrose*. It has been known from the earliest historic times. Some early writers spoke of it as "honey made from reeds without bees."

According to Albertus Agnensis, as stated by Muspratt, in the time of the Crusades sweet honeyed canes were found in great quantity in the meadows near Tripoli in Syria, which reeds were called *zucra*. The plant was cultivated, and when ripe it was bruised in mortars, the strained juice set by in vessels "till concreted in the form of snow, or white salt; this when scraped they mix with bread, or rub it in water and take it as pottage, and it is to them more wholesome and pleasing than the honey of bees."

In Europe it was used only in medicine until about the fifteenth century, and it was not produced in large quantities till about 1800.

The sucrose of commerce is also obtained from the beet, the palm, and the maple tree, and from another grass, *Sorghum saccharatum*. The process of manufacture is essentially the same in all cases, and only that of cane sugar will be referred to.

The sugar cane contains about eighteen per cent of sugar; but since about four per cent remains in the refuse from pressing, and some is lost by skimming during the boiling, and two or three per cent goes into the molasses which is the result of the boiling, there remains only from eight to twelve per cent of sugar which is recovered. The canes are crushed and passed through powerful presses. The juice is boiled with a little milk of lime, added to neutralize the acids which the juice contains: this forms a scum, which is taken off. After the boiling in vacuum pans has concentrated the juice sufficiently, it is run into a large vessel to crystallize.

The mass of crystals formed is drained from the syrup, and is known as raw or muscovado sugar. The non-crystallized portion is known as molasses. The old West India or New Orleans molasses, which made such good gingerbread, was of this type, and was somewhat acid, owing to the presence of acetic and formic acids.

The raw sugar is sent to the refineries to be made into the pure white sugar known as loaf, granulated, or powdered. The raw sugar is dissolved and boiled with the white of egg, or with the serum of blood; formerly a small quantity of chemicals, as tin salts, was sometimes used, but metallic salts are not now employed for this purpose. This boiling separates all the remaining gum, albumen, etc., and, after filtering, the juice is clear. The final filtering is through boneblack, in order to take out the color. The juice is now colorless, and after boiling in vacuum pans is allowed to cool and crystallize. Some sugar is rendered non-crystallizable by this last boiling, and this is known as syrup. The *golden syrup* among others should be from this product; in England the crude syrup is called *treacle*. With the improved processes of boiling in vacuum pans the old molasses has almost disappeared, and syrups have become more costly. Much of the old time molasses went to the distilleries, to be made into rum. The grades of sugar have also changed very much. The dark brown sugars have almost disappeared from the market. This is owing to the improved methods of boiling. The granulated is of the same quality as loaf sugar, only the syrup is stirred while crystallizing, so that the crystals do not cohere. The light brown sugars are the next product, containing some molasses, and therefore they taste sweeter, since the flavor is more pronounced in the colored portion of the juice.

If the granulated sugar is not quite freed from the syrup, it tastes more decidedly sweet than if it is perfectly pure. That is, it has more the taste which we are accustomed to associate with sugar.

It is often said that powdered sugar must be adulterated, because it does not sweeten as much as loaf sugar; but such is not the case, and some explanation must be sought. The reason seems to be twofold: first, a spoonful of powdered sugar does not weigh as much as a spoonful of granulated; secondly, since sweetness is a physical property, the finely divided condition of the sugar has something to do with it. The coarser grains seem to excite in the nerves of taste a stronger vibration, so to speak, in dissolving, than do the fine particles. To prove this, equal weights of loaf, of granulated of different degrees of fineness, of powdered, and of coffee-crushed sugar, were dissolved in equal volumes of water, and then tested by various persons, the tumblers containing the solutions being numbered so that the taster was an unbiased judge. Some pure honey was added to the list, and the results confirmed the previous suspicions that the taste was not due to the chemical purity of the substance. In every case the coffee sugar was pronounced the sweetest, and that of the solution of honey the least sweet. As to the solutions of the other sugars, which were all pure sucrose, judgments varied, showing that the sensation of sweetness is not owing solely to the presence of a certain amount of sucrose.

That beet root contained a sugar identical with that obtained from the sugar cane was first made known by Margraf, in 1747. But the beet was not cultivated for the purpose to any extent until the middle of this century. Under the protection of Napoleon I., the industry gradually gained ground. A prize of a million francs was offered for the successful manufacture of sugar from plants of home growth. As late as 1860 the fate of beet sugar was doubtful, since the disagreeable flavor of the molasses still clung to the crystallized sugar. But applied science has overcome all the difficulties, and the purest loaf sugar is now made from beets. About one third of the total sugar product is beet-root sugar. In 1858, the amount of beet sugar produced was estimated at 159,821 tons; in 1878, at 1,420,800 tons for Europe alone. The culture of the beet has spread throughout Germany and Russia. It has been tried in England, Ireland, and the Northern United States; and it doubtless will prove a source of profit in many latitudes where the sugar cane will not thrive. Beets contain up to ten or twelve per cent of sugar. In Belgium and France they extract about seven per cent, and in Germany eight or nine per cent. The process of manufacture differs little from that of cane sugar. The molasses from beet sugar is mostly sent to the distillery, as there is a very disagreeable taste to it.

In parts of the United States and in Canada sugar is made from the sap of the maple, *Acer saccharinum*, and other allied species. The sugar is cane sugar, or sucrose, and the accompanying substances in the sap give an agreeable flavor quite peculiar to maple sugar. Several million pounds are annually produced.

The cultivation of the Chinese sugar grass, or sugar millet, (*Sorghum saccharatum*,) has been recently attempted in the United States, with some success. It seems to be suited to a warm temperate zone, and thus is intermediate between the Northern maple and beet and the tropical sugar cane.

Grape sugar (so called from its abundance in that fruit, some ten to fifteen per cent) is found in a great variety of fruits. Apples contain eight per cent, strawberries five or six per cent, cranberries and gooseberries seven per cent, blackberries and raspberries four per cent, peaches and plums one to two per cent. It is present in the sacs of flowers and is the source of honey. It can be readily obtained from grapes by expressing the juice, and, after neutralization of the acids, the syrup may be refined and crystallized as in the case of beet sugar, but is then apt to take on water and become moist. It is accompanied by a difficultly crystallizable sugar called *levulose*. Grape sugar made from grapes is too costly for ordinary use. Two processes for its cheap production are employed, but for the understanding of these a short statement of the changes which cane sugar may undergo will be necessary. Sucrose ($C_{12}H_{22}O_{11}$), when boiled for a length of time in contact with air, and especially if acid be present, becomes changed into *invert sugar*, as it is called, from its behavior when a beam of polarized light is passed through it. This invert sugar can be separated into two kinds: dextrose ($C_6H_{12}O_6$), a crystallizable sugar turning the ray of polarized light to the right, identical with the sugar obtained from grapes; and a difficultly crystallizable sugar turning the ray of polarized light to the left, and which from this property is called levulose, or fruit sugar ($C_6H_{12}O_6$). Thus its chemical composition is identical with dextrose. Both kinds are often called *glucose*, meaning sweet, from the Greek *glukus*. In jellies and preserved fruits, a large portion of the cane sugar or sucrose is changed into glucose during the heating with the acid juice of the fruit, and, as was noticed, molasses is chiefly the invert sugar caused by boiling the acid juice of the sugar cane. But not only may sucrose be converted into glucose, but all forms of starch ($C_6H_{10}O_5$) may, by the action of two kinds of agents, be changed into glucose ($C_6H_{12}O_6$). One of these agents is the diastase or starch converter, a ferment found in sprouting grain. By this means beer, bread, etc. are made. The sugar thus formed is called *maltose*. It is an intermediate sugar, having the composition of cane sugar, but it reduces copper sulphate, which cane sugar does not. This process is not available for obtaining clean sugar, since the various other ingredients of the potato or grain used are in the mash; also a portion of the sugar will be lost by the further change into alcohol; hence, for the manufacture of commercial glucose, the starch is usually obtained first, and afterward boiled with very dilute acid for some hours. The intermediate products dextrine and maltose are formed as well as dextrose, the relative amounts dependent upon the time of boiling. The acid is then neutralized, usually with lime. Where sulphuric acid is used a little of the calcium sulphate, being slightly soluble in water, will be found in the syrup or sugar. Hence the stories of free sulphuric acid in glucose. The concentration and refining are then conducted as for cane sugar. A bushel of corn will give thirty-two pounds of glucose. Twenty establishments in the United States can make 609,000,000 pounds annually.

All woody fibre or cellulose ($C_6H_{10}O_5$) can be acted upon by acids so as to form glucose; hence any woody substance, as sawdust, cotton, etc., can be converted, by the addition of molecules of water, into glucose; but this is not done for the purpose of sugar manufacture, corn meal being much more available. For spirits it has probably been done. The proper name of glucose should be *starch sugar*.

Properties of Glucose.

Glucose is one and a half times less soluble than sucrose, or it requires one and a third times its weight of cold water to dissolve it. It requires two and a half times more of grape sugar to sweeten the same volume of water than it does of cane sugar; hence, while it is cheaper, it is not as valuable, pound for pound.

Glucose as it is usually sold contains about twenty per cent of water and about twenty per cent of unfermentable substances, leaving only some sixty per cent of sugar, although the sugar may run as high as seventy-five per cent. The syrups contain from thirty to forty per cent of sugar. Honey is essentially glucose, or dextrose, with perhaps some levulose, and something not sugar, to which no name has yet been given. The proportion of non-fermentable substances varies according to the source of the honey. Sometimes as much as fifteen per cent is found.

The following is a summary of the report on glucose made by the Committee of the National Academy of Sciences to the Commissioner of Internal Revenue, in 1884: —

"1. Starch sugar as found in commerce is a mixture in varying proportions of two sugars called dextrose and maltose, and of dextrine or starch gum. Dextrose was discovered in grapes by Lowitz in 1792, and was first prepared from starch by Kirchhoff in 1811. In 1819, Braconnot prepared it from woody fibre. Maltose was first recognized as a distinct sugar by Dubremfant in 1847, in the product of the action of malt on starch. No dextrose is thus produced, according to O'Sullivan.

"2. The process of making starch sugar consists, first, in separating the starch from the corn by soaking, grinding, straining, and settling; and second in converting the starch into sugar by the action of dilute sulphuric acid, this acid being subsequently removed by the action of chalk. To make the solid 'grape sugar' the conversion is carried further than to make liquid 'glucose.' After clarifying, the liquid is concentrated in vacuum pans and is decolorized with bone-black.

"3. The starch sugar industry in the United States gives employment to twenty-nine factories, having an estimated capital of $5,000,000, consuming about 40,000 bushels of corn per day, and producing grape sugar and glucose to the annual value of nearly $10,000,000. In Germany in 1881–82 there were thirty-nine factories of this sort, consuming over 70,000 tons of starch, and producing about 40,000 tons of starch sugar.

"4. Starch sugar is chiefly used in making table syrup, in brewing beer as substitute for malt, and in adulterating cane sugar. It is also used to replace cane sugar in confectionery, in canning fruits, in making fruit jellies, and in cooking. Artificial honey is made with it, and so also is vinegar.

"5. Starch sugar represents one distinct class of sugar, as cane sugar does the other, the former being obtained naturally from the grape, as the latter is from the cane and the beet. Starch sugar, which is a term chemically synonymous with dextrose and glucose, when pure, has about two thirds the sweetening power of sugar cane. By the action of the dilute acids both cane sugar and starch yield dextrose. In the case of starch, however, dextrose constitutes the sole final product.

"6. The commercial samples of starch sugar obtained by the committee showed a fairly uniform composition on analysis. The liquid form, or 'glucose,' contained from 34.3 to 42.8 per cent of dextrose, from 0 to 19.3 per cent of maltose, from 29.8 to 45.3 per cent of dextrine, and from 14.2 to 22.6 per cent of water. The solid form, grape sugar, gave from 72 to 73.4 per cent of dextrose, from 0 to 36 per cent of maltose, from 4.3 to 9.1 per cent of dextrine, and from 14 to 17.6 per cent of water. Three specimens of especially prepared 'grape sugar' contained 87.1, 93.2, and 99.4 per cent of dextrose respectively. The last of these was crystalline anhydrous dextrose.

"7. Of mineral or inorganic constituents, the samples of starch sugar examined contained only minute quantities. The total ash formed in the 'glucose' was only from 0.325 to 1.000 per cent, and in the 'grape sugars' only from 0.335 to 0.750 per cent. No impurities, either organic or inorganic in character, other than those mentioned, were detected in any of the samples examined.

"In conclusion, then, the following facts appear as the result of the present investigation : —

"(1.) That the manufacture of sugar from starch is a long-established industry, scientifically valuable and commercially important.

"(2.) That the processes which it employs at the present time are unobjectionable in their character, and leave the product uncontaminated.

"(3.) That starch sugar thus made and sent into commerce is of exceptional purity and uniformity of composition, and contains no injurious substances; and,

"(4.) That, though having at best only about two thirds the sweetening power of cane sugar, yet starch sugar is in no way inferior to cane sugar in healthfulness, there being no evidence before the committee that maize starch sugar, either in its normal condition or fermented, has any deleterious effect upon the system, even when taken in large quantities."

The report is signed by George F. Barker, Chairman, William H. Brewer, Charles F. Chandler, Wolcott Gibbs, and Ira Remsen.

Uses of Sugar.

Taking the world as a whole, it might be said that sugar was used as a condiment rather than as a food, but in the light of recent statistics it seems a very important article of diet, and should be so considered. Its use seems to be steadily on the increase. In Great Britain in 1700 the total yearly consumption was only 10,000 pounds. In 1867 it was 44.15 pounds per head; while in 1876 it had reached 63 pounds, and in 1884, 67 pounds. An estimate from the statistics of 1867, reckoned by races, gave the consumption of sugar per head as 41.40 pounds for the Anglo-Saxon races, 12.34 for the Latin, 7.30 for the Teutonic, and 3.30 for Russia, Turkey, and Greece. In the United States in 1875 it was 44 pounds, in 1884, 56 pounds, and in 1896, 62 pounds per head, making the total consumption for 1896 nearly four billions of pounds. It would seem that in the North it is taking the place of the oil of the South as a heat-giving food. The growing opinion seems to be in favor of its moderate use. It is true that, if the stomach is not able to digest it at once, it is liable to change into lactic acid, instead of being absorbed into the system. This only shows that sugar is not suitable for that individual at that time. The very general craving for sweets is undoubtedly founded on a law of demand of the system. Like all other foods, sugar may be abused. That it plays a part as a heat-giving food is indicated by the fact that it is not craved to so great an extent in summer as in winter. Hence a moderate use of it by children is not to be rashly condemned.

The changes which sugar undergoes in the system are not fully understood, yet it is pretty certain that cane sugar, sucrose, is not absorbed as such, but is converted into glucose before it is assimilated. With this in view, it seems difficult to prove the oft-repeated assertion of the opponents of artificial sugar, that it is injurious. As we have seen, there are several kinds of sugar included under the general term of glucose, and just what the physiological properties of each of these kinds are we do not yet know; but the burden of proof lies with those who assert the unwholesomeness of glucose. It has never been supposed that the sometimes poisonous properties of honey were due to the sugar, but to the pollen or other matters obtained from the flowers by the bees.

The adulteration of sugar may be considered under three heads. First, the addition of insoluble substances, such as marble dust, which is sometimes found advertised among the supplies of confectioners. It is said that sand used to be added. Second, the foreign substances left in from the process of manufacture, such as ultramarine to give the requisite blue color. If tin were ever found in sugar, it would be in this list. Third, and most frequent at present, is the addition of glucose or corn sugar, which is much cheaper, but is less sweet, partly on account of its lesser solubility in water. One quart of water dissolves three pounds of cane sugar, but only one or one and a half pounds of grape sugar.

Sugar may be so manipulated in refining as to be white and crystalline, and yet contain quite a percentage of moisture and syrup. Such sugar cakes together on standing. The presence of this moisture may be regarded as an adulteration.

The adulteration of the granulated and powdered sugars, at least those sold in the Eastern States, is not as extensive as has been supposed. Of the samples examined by the writer, not one of seventy-three samples from Massachusetts, not one of five from New York, and only one of twelve from Chicago, was adulterated.

The Report of the New York State Board of Health of 1882 gives one hundred and sixteen samples examined. In no case was there any intentional addition of insoluble mineral matter. Of the thirty-three powdered sugars, none were adulterated. Of the sixty-seven brown sugars, four were mixed with glucose.

The tests are not very difficult as to the presence of foreign matters, since they are insoluble in water, and half a pound of sugar dissolved in a pint of water will leave a sediment if marble or sand has been added. Tin would be detected best by the battery, a plate of copper being used as a cathode, on which tin shows very quickly. The use of sulphuretted hydrogen is not to be relied upon, since on heating there seems to be formed an organic compound of the color of tin sulphide which is very misleading.

For glucose, the test with Fehling's solution is the one most used. But here care must be taken, for, as has been said, sucrose on heating changes to invert sugar, which reduces the copper of the solution; so that the mere fact of a slight reduction of copper does not prove wilful adulteration. For instance, in the case of candies, the writer has never yet been able to find candy or confectionery which did not reduce Fehling's solution; but it is by no means to be concluded that all confectionery is made from glucose, although undoubtedly a large part of it is so made.

Dietzsch (page 277) gives the following as a qualitative test. A dilute solution of sugar is colored skyblue with a few drops of Fehling's solution, and heated to the boiling point. If the sugar is all cane sugar, the liquid may stand twenty-four hours without showing any change; but if glucose or invert sugar is present, the reddish color of the reduced copper oxide will appear in a few minutes.

Fehling's solution may be made as follows: 34.632 grams of pure dry copper sulphate are dissolved in 500 cc. of water and put into a bottle with a glass stopper. 173 grams of Rochelle salt — tartrate of sodium and ammonium — and 125 grams of potassium hydrate are dissolved in 500 cc. of water, and put into a bottle with a rubber stopper. A glass stopper will be liable to become fastened in the bottle containing caustic alkalies. The solution of copper will preserve its strength much longer if kept separate from the alkaline liquid. For use, mix the two in equal proportions, measuring the copper accurately. 50 cc. of the copper, or 100 of the mixture, are considered to reduce .5 gram of grape or of invert sugar.

The skilled analyst uses the polariscope or saccharimeter to determine the percentage of pure sugar. (See Blyth, page 120.)

A simple method of detecting starch sugar in the presence of cane sugar has been proposed by P. Casamajor. The suspected sugar is thoroughly dried, then treated with methyl-alcohol which has been saturated with starch sugar. 100 cc. of methyl-alcohol of 50° strength dissolves about 57 grams of starch sugar, and will not take up any more, but will readily dissolve cane sugar, thus taking it out of a mixture, leaving the adulterant undissolved.

The presence of dextrine in syrups may be detected by adding an equal volume of strong alcohol to the undiluted syrup. The dextrine will be precipitated as a white gelatinous mass.

Syrups are very liable to be *not* what they seem. Dr. Kedzie, of Michigan, in 1879, found only one out of twenty-one genuine. The black color sometimes noticed when syrup is put into tea is due to the presence of the salts of iron derived from the pans during boiling.

HONEY.

It is reported that over 63,000,000 pounds of honey were produced in the United States in 1889, more than one-tenth of this coming from Iowa.

It is said, especially by English analysts, that much American honey is entirely artificial, the comb being made of paraffine and filled with glucose syrup. Two simple tests will show whether this is the case. Normal honey, being collected by the bees from flowers, will contain many pollen grains. The absence of these is a suspicious circumstance. Beeswax is blackened by warm sulphuric acid, while paraffine is not affected.

VI.

CANNED FRUITS AND MEATS, OR TINNED GOODS.

IF an ordinary tin fruit-can is opened, and its inner surface examined, it will be found covered with the crystalline figures often produced by the action of dilute acids upon tin, and known as "moirée métallique." This apparent corrosion of the metallic surface suggests the possibility that an acid fruit, if kept for a sufficient time in such a can, may take into solution an injurious quantity of metallic impurity. Moreover, in the making and sealing of cans, a greater or less amount of solder finds its way inside, and thus the fruit comes in contact with an alloy containing from thirty to sixty per cent of lead. All the common fruits — the tomato, peach, plum, cherry, apple, pear, currant, etc. — owe their acidity to the presence of acid malates, malic acid, or other organic acids.

Considerable excitement is caused every now and then by newspaper stories of the presence of tin in canned foods, and of the illnesses thus caused. In England, especially, the chemists have paid considerable attention to the subject; and although there is an objection to the calculation of the tin as stannous hydrate, the results are interesting.

Mr. Wynter Blyth tested canned fruits (apricots, tomatoes, etc.), and in twenty-three samples the amounts found, calculated as stannous hydrate, ranged from 1.9 to 14.3 grains per pound, the mean amount being 5.2 grains. The juice and fruit, in some instances, had a metallic taste. Several of the tins showed signs of corrosion.

The Journal of the Society of Arts says: "The little that is known of the action of stannous hydrate may be summed up in a few lines. Doses of about .174 gram per kilo, of body weight, cause, in guinea-pigs, death, with signs of intestinal irritation; but with doses smaller than .17 to .2 gram, the effects are uncertain, and the animals usually recover. Hence, supposing a man to be affected in the same manner and proportion, he would have to consume at a meal ten pounds of the most contaminated of these tinned fruits. But it is not a question of immediate deadliness; it is rather an inquiry as to the action of small repeated doses continued for a long time."

On the latter point we have the opinions of Professor Attfield, given in an address before the London Pharmaceutical Society, in March, 1884. He had recently examined sixteen samples. He found rather less tin than Mr. Blyth. The greatest amount was in apricots and tomatoes, namely, .028 grain in a pound. The largest quantity which the speaker ever found in any food was in some canned soup containing a good deal of lemon juice; this was .03 grain in half a pint, as sent to the table. The conclusions of Professor Attfield are as follows: —

"1. I have never been able to satisfy myself that a can of ordinary tinned food contains even a useful medicinal dose of such a true soluble compound of tin as is likely to have any effect on man.

"2. As for the metal itself, — that is, the filings or actual metallic particles or fragments, — one ounce is a common dose as a vermifuge, harmless even in that quantity to man, and not always so harmful as could be desired to the parasites for whose disestablishment it is administered. One ounce might be contained in four hundred-weight of food.

" 3. If a possible harmful quantity of a soluble compound of tin be placed in a portion of canned food, the latter will be so nasty — so metallic, in fact — that no sane person will eat it.

" 4. Unsoundness in meat does not appear to promote the corrosion or solution of tin. I have kept salmon in cans until it was putrid, testing it occasionally for tin; no trace was detected. Nevertheless, food should not be allowed to remain for a few days, or even hours, in sauce-pans, metal baking-pans, or opened tin cans; for in this case it may taste metallic.

" 5. Unsound food, canned or uncanned, may of course injure health; and where canned food has really done harm, the harm has in all probability been due to the food, and not to the can.

" In my opinion, given after well weighing all evidence hitherto forthcoming, the public have not the faintest cause for alarm respecting the occurrence of tin, lead, or any other metal, in canned foods. If persons are unwise enough to let the food remain long in an opened tin can, they almost deserve to be punished by the metallic flavor which may be imparted to the food."

A late investigation by F. P. Hall, in the " Journal

of the American Chemical Society" (Vol. IV. p. 440), shows that acetic, tartaric, and citric acids corrode tin and lead when the metals are pure and when they are alloyed, but that this corrosion goes on very much more rapidly when air is admitted; that is, when the surface of the metal can become oxidized. The acetic acid dissolved about six times as much metal in the open air as in closed vessels. Cans which had been emptied of their contents were partly filled with the above-named acids. At the end of two weeks the cans which contained tartaric and citric acids respectively had given up all the tinned surface; the acetic seemed not to have acted as readily, but there was probably more solder in the other two.

The fear has been common that tin plate might be contaminated with lead. Mr. Hall's investigation seems to allay such fears. He says: "The tin plate used in this country is entirely imported, most of it coming from England. The two principal kinds are 'bright plate' and 'terne plate.' Bright plate is, or should be, tinned only with pure tin. Terne plate, often called lead plate, is known to contain large quantities of lead; it is used chiefly for roofing." He examined many samples, both of the plate as imported and of tin cans and tin-plate goods, among them those from the five-cent stores, without finding an appreciable amount of lead. The best of tin may contain traces, as it is almost impossible to obtain absolutely pure metal by any metallurgical process. The solder is then the only objection worth considering, and much more care is taken in sealing the cans than formerly. Of the tin-foil used to enwrap moist foods and yeast, the report is not so good. Of twelve samples examined which were obtained from importers, only three were pure tin, and three were nearly pure lead. Eight samples taken from food and yeast were examined. Four were pure tin; the two found on yeast were pure tin. This corresponds with the experience of the laboratory through a term of years. The two found on Neuchâtel cheese were both about three fourths lead. Of the three on chocolate two were good, while an embossed foil on a fashionable chocolate consisted of eighty per cent of lead. The use of lead-foil on cheese is objectionable.

The preservation of food means permanent sterilization. Late bacteriological experiments upon canned goods, notably clams, lobsters, and corn, seem to prove that "spoiling" is always due to a lack of sterilization. This may mean too low a degree of heat, the heat not long enough continued, or carelessness in sealing after sterilization. Long continued heating darkens certain food materials, and as the dark color is by some deemed objectionable, there is a temptation to use too low a degree of heat, or to shorten the time of heating. Those methods which ensure an actual temperature of 250 F. inside and outside for at least 10 minutes give very satisfactory results. Of one hundred cans heated in this manner not one spoiled in a month's time, although kept very warm. As the cans are sealed while hot, a vacuum is usually formed when the contents cool. This vacuum plays no part in the sterilization, but aids in the inspection. The spoiled cans commonly show a swelling upon the ends, caused by the fermentation of the contents; the sound cans have level or slightly concave ends. In purchasing, every can should be examined for this appearance, and also for any evidence of leakage.

VII.

CONDIMENTS.

MUSTARD.

THE mustard of commerce is the seed of the plant *Sinapis*, of different species, ground into flour. It belongs to one of the most useful families of our temperate zone. This is the Mustard family, Cruciferæ. It is a hardy plant, and grows very readily in our climate. The famous Durham mustard was originally made from the wild charlock, *Sinapis arvensis*, which grew abundantly around Durham, and has a pleasant, mildly pungent flavor. The name is still retained as a trade-mark. The charlock grows as a weed in our fields, but has never been here utilized. Along the coast of Ireland, the fields, as seen from the passing steamer, look yellow with the blossoms of the wild charlock, or Charlie, as it is familiarly called. Black and white mustard are the two kinds usually found in the market, — the seeds of *Sinapis nigra* and

Sinapis alba. Since the whole seeds are to be had, the best way to study the condiment is to purchase some seeds, and grind them. Several points of difference between this undoubtedly pure article, and that which is bought ground will be noticed. In the first place the ground seeds are very oily. This is not the pungent volatile oil which gives the flavor, but a bland fixed oil which is always expressed from the seeds before they are manufactured into mustard. It finds a ready sale as a lubricant, and is said to enter largely into the composition of cosmoline, etc., forming the basis of these emollients, to which petroleum is then added.

Next, the color of the pure mustard will attract attention. There is no mustard of a bright yellow color, the brightest possible color being a dull yellow. The bright yellow of the shops, is either largely rape-seed, or artificially colored to suit a popular taste. Another noticeable difference is in the pungent smell and taste of the home-ground article. If such mustard is used for a time, that of the shops seems very insipid.

Mustard is one of the most universal and wholesome condiments, but its use in medicine is even more important. It is of the utmost consequence to have a genuine article, when it is to be used as an active remedy in sudden illness. The balance of life and death may depend upon the quality of the mustard used for the emetic, the plaster, or the bath. Every housekeeper should see that her medicine-chest is supplied with pure mustard, whatever may be the quality of that in her spice-box.

The adulterations are many. Probably two thirds of the mustard sold is anything but pure ground seeds. The principal ingredients are starch from wheat, rice, or corn flour, tumeric to color the too white starch, rape-seed, old turnip and radish seed unfit for planting, linseed, etc.

Of the thirty samples examined in the laboratory of the writer, twenty-one contained more or less starch. Hardly any seeds of Cruciferæ contain starch; hence its presence is a proof of adulteration. The blue or dark-purple color which iodine causes in starch grains, and the thickening in boiling water, are the simplest tests. In eleven samples tumeric was added. This was readily detected by the microscope, as are also the other seeds. The per cent of oil may be used to determine the relative strengths of a number of samples, since it is upon the volatile, pungent oil that the peculiar properties of mustard depend. In 1882, Professor Lattimore found sixty-six per cent of the samples examined for the New York State Board of Health to be adulterated. The addition of any mineral matter, such as terra-alba, yellow ochre, etc., may be detected by burning two or three grams, and weighing the ash. The genuine mustard gives about four per cent of ash.

PEPPER.

Pepper-corns are the berries of the plant *Piper nigrum*, which grows only in tropical climates. Hassall says that Malabar, Penang, and Sumatra are the three kinds most prized. Black and white pepper are from the same plant, the only difference being that black pepper is the whole berry, while the white has been deprived of the husk or outer layer of the berry, which is black. White pepper is milder than the black, for the husks are quite pungent. The best is that from the whole berry. A good way to secure pure pepper is to use a little mill on the table, and to grind the whole berries as wanted. The mills are now to be had, imported from Europe. The active properties of pepper depend upon three substances, — about sixteen per cent of acrid resin and piperine, and one to two per cent of volatile oil.

The adulteration of pepper is extensive. Indeed, it is the exception, rather than the rule, to find a pure article in the market. Wheat flour, ground rice, Indian meal, husks of the London-made white pepper, husks of mustard, and the mysterious "P. D." pepper dust, said to be the sweepings of the warehouses, can be imported for as many cents a pound as the prepared article can be sold for per ounce ; so that there is great temptation to use these harmless, but not tempting mixtures. Time and trouble are saved by the purchase of ready-ground condiments, but the price paid is too great in proportion.

Of sixteen samples examined, three were fairly good ; nine were made up of pepper and mustard husks, flour, and Indian meal. Most of the adulterations can be detected by the microscope, after a careful study of the structure of the various seeds and husks ; but experience has taught the writer, that considerable practice is required to become expert at the detection of the kind of foreign matters used. The result of the examination of pepper, under the direction of the New York State Board of Health in 1882 showed that seventy per cent of the commercial article was adulterated.

Cayenne Pepper.

Red or Cayenne pepper is made from the ground pods of various species of Capsicum, a plant of the Nightshade family. The cayenne of commerce is derived from tropical species, but the pods of the red peppers which are commonly cultivated for pickles, when ground, make a very good cayenne. The peculiar pungent taste is due to the presence of about four per cent of an acrid resin. The earlier English writers state that cayenne is more liable to adulteration than black pepper, and alarming stories are told of the presence of red-lead, mercury, etc. But the results of examinations made in this country do not show any poisonous addition, and the addition of flour, etc., is rather less than in black pepper.

SPICES.

Those spices, like nutmeg, cloves, stick cinnamon, mace, and allspice, which are bought by weight, and in the form in which they are gathered, are not exactly capable of adulteration. But there is a certain deception to be guarded against. An inferior or cheaper quality of the same or of a similar kind of spice may be mixed with, or substituted for, better or more costly sorts, without any corresponding diminution in price.

For instance, wild nutmegs are mixed with cultivated ones, bearing about the same relation to the best qualities that a cider apple does to a fine Baldwin. It is the same with mace and cloves, while cassia is substituted for cinnamon only too largely, so that it is almost impossible to find stick cinnamon that is not mixed with cassia. To learn to know the genuine species with certainty, is our only safeguard. Then, if we choose to buy cassia, we shall do it with our eyes open, and without paying the price of the delicate and costly cinnamon.

Nutmegs.

There are three species of Myristica which furnish nutmegs. The best are the kernels of the *Myristica fragrans*, and are called queen nutmegs. The tree is a native of the East India islands, but is also cultivated in India and Central America. The best nutmegs are those from Penang, which are about an inch in length, shaped like a damson plum. The kernels are usually pickled in lime-water, to ward off the attacks of insects to which they are particularly liable. The weight of good nutmegs should be, on an average, one hundred to the pound, or nearly seven to the ounce, grocers' weight. Very fine ones weigh eighty and one hundred to the pound, or five or six to the ounce. If pricked with a pin, the oil exudes visibly, and the pin also penetrates readily. Wild nutmegs are small and pointed. They are inferior in the amount of oil, and in the general fragrance.

Cinnamon.

The best cinnamon comes from Ceylon. It is the bark of a tree of the Laurel family, which gives us, even in this temperate climate, such plants as our sassafras and our spice-bush. The trees are topped like osier willows, and the cinnamon used is the bark from the young shoots, which form the bush at the top of the tree, and which are cut twice a year. A tract not much more than a quarter of a mile square forms the great cinnamon orchard of Ceylon. No other country produces so fine a quality, or so great a quantity, as the fertile and siliceous tracts of Ceylon and the neighboring islands.

The most noticeable character of true cinnamon is its splintery, fibrous quality. It tears rather than breaks, and is in small, thin rolls. The taste is sweet and spicy, and it retains its flavor long in the mouth. *Cassia*, or *Chinese cinnamon*, is used to mix with it, being cheap and abundant. It is coarser and in thicker rolls It breaks readily, but does not tear, and if chewed is granular and rather mucilaginous. It lacks the delicate, sweet taste and smell of cinnamon, having a peculiar woody, strong flavor of its own.

The amount of true cinnamon consumed in the United States for the year ending June 30, 1875, was valued at $4,013, while the value of cassia was $279,250, or nearly seventy times as much.

Mace.

Mace is the aril of the nutmeg, and its quality depends very greatly upon the kind of kernel upon which it grows, the aril of the queen nutmeg being the best.

Cloves.

Cloves are the unexpanded flower-buds of the *Caryophyllus aromaticus*, a tree of the Myrtle family, which is a native of the Moluccas, but which is cultivated in the East and West Indies, Guiana, and Brazil. Like all the spices under consideration, the active principle is due to one or more oils, which may be, and are, extracted and sold as oil of clove, oil of cassia, etc. Whole cloves can hardly be said to be adulterated, although the stalks are sometimes in excess of the buds, and advantage is taken of the property of imbibing a large portion of moisture to increase the weight.

Pimento, or Allspice.

Pimento is the berry of the *Euginia pimento*, a tree of the Myrtle family, a native of the Caribbee Islands, and also cultivated in the East Indies. The berries have a fragrant odor, supposed to resemble a mixture of cloves, cinnamon, and nutmegs: hence the name of Allspice.

Ginger.

The ginger plant, *Zinziber officinale,* belongs to the order from which tumeric and East India arrow-root are obtained. It is a native of India and China, and is cultivated in Tropical America and Africa. The ginger of commerce is derived from the fleshy creeping root-stalks, which are dug up when about a year old, and, if scraped and dried, give white or Jamaica ginger; if left coated, or unscraped, black or East India ginger. Calcutta exports the principal part of the ginger used. Ginger contains, besides the volatile oil, an aromatic resin.

Curry.

Curry is not very extensively used in America, yet it is found so often as to justify a word. It is composed of a mixture of spices, and highly colored with tumeric. It is liable to variations of strength, as are the spices of which it is composed.

Adulteration of Spices.

In ground spices, as a rule, we find much reason for dissatisfaction. Their only merit now is convenience, not quality. Nutmegs, mace, and cloves are so oily that, to grind them easily, some absorbent like sawdust or starch is added, and this becomes a part of the ground spice as the first step, whatever may be added later. There is, however, but little demand for ground nutmeg, American housekeepers having the good sense to prefer the whole nuts.

Twelve specimens of cinnamon were examined. Only three of these contained any cinnamon at all. Even these were mixed with cassia and sawdust. The other nine were chiefly cassia and sawdust, mahogany sawdust being distinctly identified in some of them. Two contained a very little cassia and a great deal of sawdust; and the third was nothing but sawdust, there being no trace of any spice in it.

Professor Lattimore, in the New York State Board of Health Report for 1883, found that of the samples examined seventy per cent of the allspice was adulterated, eighty-two per cent of the cinnamon, fifty-seven per cent of the cassia, seventy-six per cent of the cloves; but no poisonous substance was found in any.

All these spices may be examined under the microscope for adulterations; but, as has been said before, experience only will give the training of the eye which will render an opinion worth anything. Each kind of spice here mentioned has its own peculiarities, and, after these are thoroughly studied, the additions may be at once determined. The adulterations are much the same in all this class, — starch in some form, tumeric for color, mustard husks for pungency. Professor Lattimore gives the per cent of adulteration of the fifteen gingers which he examined as sixty-six, but the samples from Boston and vicinity seem better. Of twenty-eight specimens, only seven (or twenty-five per cent) were adulterated. Three of these were adulterated with starch and tumeric, one with starch and mustard husks, one with tumeric, and two with starch only. The remaining twenty-one varied in color from a tawny white to brown, but were all fragrant and good, and some excellent. None were at all yellow, except the four to which tumeric had been added. The difference in color is owing simply to the preparation. The bark is scraped off the fleshy roots, as in the whole white ginger-root, or the preserved ginger. Then the ground ginger is quite light in color. If the bark is left on, the ginger is brown when ground. In whole ginger there is often a white coating upon the roots. This is only lime, into which they have been dipped to protect them from insects.

SALAD OIL.

Some other condiments deserve a passing notice. Among these may be classed salad oil, which has until recently been olive oil of various grades, but all expressed from the fruit of the olive tree. But as the demand grew, and as the American refined lard oil became cheap, great quantities are said to have been shipped to the oil-producing countries of Italy, and returned in the shape of pure olive. It has been supposed that certain grades of refined petroleum oils have been used for the same purpose, though the exportation was very carefully managed. At present a great deal of the salad oil has never crossed the seas, but is known to the dealers for what it is, cotton-seed oil. The oil is pressed out from the cotton seeds by powerful presses, and makes a very clear, sweet oil, just as wholesome, for aught any one knows, as the oil pressed from the olive, and for home use it is certainly much cheaper. The trouble with the sale of it being, like that of oleomargarine, that it is sold under false pretences, and for an exorbitant price.

The detection of the per cent of cotton-seed oil in the presence of olive oil is difficult, and the presence of lard oil is likewise very hard to determine, so that it is of little use to give here the various tests which have been proposed. The chemistry of the several oils is not understood sufficiently to allow of definite statements, and since the chemical composition of the oils, so far as it is known, shows them to be similar, it is a question if it will be possible to separate the elements of the seed oils with the same certainty that one metallic element is separated from another.

FLAVORING EXTRACTS.

These have had, periodically, highly sensational stories told about them. In the two or three dozen samples examined in the laboratory, no harmful ingredient was found. There was a great deal of difference in the strength of the different brands. Most of the lemon flavor is only dilute alcohol, in which a few drops of oil of lemon is dissolved, and there are only a few which are what the name would imply.

VINEGAR.

Vinegar, *vin aigre*, as its name implies, was originally made from sour wine, that is, from wine in which the alcoholic fermentation had given place to that which produces acetic acid. The whole of the alcohol may be changed into acetic acid by means of the vinegar ferment, *Mycodermi aceti*, commonly called *mother of vinegar*. A very little of this in the presence of air is sufficient to convert a large quantity of alcohol. The reaction seems to be as follows: common ethylic alcohol (C_2H_6O), by the addition of two atoms of oxygen, yields acetic acid and water ($H_2O + C_2H_4O_2$).

In the so-called "quick" or "German" process, the oxidation of the weak alcoholic liquor is hastened by letting it trickle through shavings already saturated with vinegar, the temperature being maintained at about 90° F.

In the United States the alcoholic liquor used is chiefly whiskey, diluted with eight or ten times its bulk of water. Tall tubs, sometimes twenty or more feet high, are filled with clean beech shavings well packed, These are first soaked with strong vinegar; then the diluted whiskey is poured on the top, a little at a time, and slowly finds its way down to the bottom, where it is drawn off as vinegar. The air is let in near the bottom by small orifices, and finds its way to the top by the draft caused by the heat of the oxidation.

Whiskey may thus be converted into vinegar in twenty-four hours.

Cider is also used to a considerable extent, in the United States, for the manufacture of vinegar. In former years, most of it was derived from this source. The cider is left for a longer time (from eight to ten months) in half-filled casks, the bungs being left out to allow the free entrance of air. The flavor of cider vinegar is peculiar, and is much preferred by many people.

Proof vinegar contains about five per cent of acetic acid, but that sold in the shops often contains only three per cent, or even less. Because of the high price of vinegar, it has frequently been adulterated with other acids, such as sulphuric, muriatic, and rarely with nitric. They may be detected as follows. To one portion of the suspected vinegar add a few drops of barium chloride. Only a slight cloudiness should appear, but any considerable precipitate will show the presence of an undue amount of sulphuric acid. Hydrochloric acid is shown by the addition of a few drops of silver nitrate to a fresh portion of the sample. A white flocculent precipitate will appear if there has been an addition of hydrochloric acid. For the relative strength of a number of samples, if the apparatus for volumetric analysis is at hand, the quantity of soda which the same number of cubic centimetres will neutralize, will give an approximate test, but not exact, because acetate of sodium has itself a slight alkaline reaction. With baryta water (barium hydrate) as the alkali, and tumeric as the test paper, the method gives very close results.

For ketchups, sauces, and pickles which are prepared with vinegar, pure vinegar should be used. In the case of pickles, a depraved taste has led to the demand for bright green pickles, and this taste has sometimes been gratified by boiling the pickles in copper kettles with vinegar and a little alum. The acetic acid of the vinegar acts upon the copper, forming a little acetate of copper, one of the most poisonous of all the salts of copper; and this, being absorbed by the pickles, colors them green. Cheap pickles are put up in adulterated vinegar. The tests are the same as those given above. For the presence of copper, immerse a strip of clean bright iron in the liquid, and, if copper is present, the iron will become coated with a thin film of metallic copper.

SALT.

Salt is of universal use, and it has been known from the earliest times. It is found in a solid rock-like form in many countries. Salt springs are not uncommon, and on the coast the evaporation of sea-water gives sea-salt. Rock-salt is mined in Austria and at Northwick, near Liverpool, in England. A mine is now worked in Louisiana. Much salt is made in New York, Michigan, Ohio, Virginia, and West Virginia, by evaporating the water of salt springs. Salt is nearly pure sodium chloride, but it almost always contains small quantities of chloride of magnesium, which causes the salt to become moist in damp air, and which gives it the bitter taste often noticed.

There is a difference of opinion as to the healthfulness of salt when taken with food. Habit, rather than common sense, seems to govern the amount used.

VIII.

PERISHABLE FOODS, AND THE MEANS FOR PRESERVING THEM.

MEAT, FISH, ETC.

SINCE butcher's *meat* is not liable to adulteration, properly speaking, any extended discussion of its character would be out of place in this little volume. Yet it cannot be passed by without a word, for it is a form of food which requires very little expenditure of force for its assimilation, since that work was done by the animal when living, and man avails himself of it. Rightly used, it forms a valuable addition to man's diet. The consumption of meat has steadily increased, in spite of the increase in price. It is said that the cost of meat in England has increased thirty-five per cent in the past twenty-two years. A large quantity of dried and tinned meat is now exported from Australia and South America.

The amount consumed in different countries varies from about one tenth of a pound a day, or one pound in ten days, in Russia and Spain, one pound in three days in England, one in two days in New York, to a pound a day in Buenos Ayres and Uruguay, where animals are killed for their hides and horns. Meat should be obtained from healthy animals, and kept in a clean place, in order that it may form a wholesome food. The bad odor of tainted meat should be a sufficient warning of its character. A very slight taint, such as sometimes occurs on the outer edges, may be corrected by placing some charcoal in the water in which it is boiling. In order to kill all parasites, meat should be thoroughly cooked; and for this, boiling is safer than roasting. A general average composition may be shown by the following mean of many analyses: —

	Mineral Matter.	Nitrogenous Substance.	Fat.	Water.
Beef	5 per ct.	15 per ct.	30 per ct.	50 per ct.
Mutton	3.5 "	12.5 "	40 "	44 "

Fish seems to be somewhat less digestible than meat, possibly on account of the little blood in the tissue. The average composition is: mineral matter, one to two per cent; nitrogenous substance, ten to twenty; fat, five to ten; water, seventy to eighty per cent.

Eggs contain all the necessary constituents of food in the most concentrated form,—so concentrated as to be unsuited for the whole of the daily ration. For convalescents they are invaluable when they can be obtained fresh. From their very composition they are extremely liable to putrefaction. This change may be prevented by the exclusion of air, either by coating the shell with an impervious layer of oil, gum, or paraffine, or by treatment with calcium salts, or by plunging the egg into boiling water for a few seconds. Desiccated eggs are now much used.

The seeds of the Leguminosæ, *peas, beans,* and *lentils,* may be called meat substitutes, since they contain about twenty-five per cent of nitrogenous substance, twelve of water, and fifty of starch. As dried seeds they should stand next in importance to the cereals; but since beans and peas especially are eaten green, as vegetables, even more than in the dried state, they cannot be omitted in this list. This form of food is not sufficiently appreciated, especially by working people. It should be eaten with starch or fat foods. Hence the New England dish of baked pork and beans was a perfectly suitable and well-proportioned food for people whose life was spent largely in the open air, in arduous pioneer work. The nutritious seeds are less easily digested than the cereals. The "ash" contains more lime and less phosphates. Some member of this group of plants grows in every land.

VEGETABLES AND FRUITS.

Vegetables are usually understood to include certain roots and tubers, as the potato, sweet potato, turnip, and beet, with some fruits, as the tomato, squash, and cucumber. These are used in the fresh condition, and are not subject to adulteration. They are largely composed of water, seventy-five to ninety five per cent. The small nutritive value which they possess is due to the starch and sugar, and not to the nitrogenous material, which is present in small quantity only. The percentage of "ash" is higher than in cereals, and contains more potassium salts. This is also the case in *fruits*, so called, — apple, pear, grape, peach, and orange. These contain sugar, instead of the starch of the vegetable, and also an acid which gives a pleasant relish and is a stimulant to the appetite. The general composition of fruits may be stated at eighty-five per cent water, eight per cent sugar, and one per cent acid. When much salted meat is eaten, fruit and vegetables are very essential correctives of diet, on account of the acid, and possibly on account of the potassium salts, which are supposed to replace the excess of sodium salts taken with the meat.

There is little danger in the use of vegetables and fruits as food, if they are fresh, not wilted, and are fully grown or ripened. The skin of the potato contains a poisonous substance, which is volatilized when the tuber is boiled, steamed, or baked. The skin of the cucumber is indigestible, as is that of the peach. Currants should be well washed before being placed upon the table, as the bushes are often dusted over with hellebore, or with Paris green, an arsenical preparation, to prevent the ravages of worms.

The same caution is applicable to some of the *relishes*, as lettuce and cabbage. These green foods should be crisp, not wilted. They are important adjuncts to diet on account of the mineral matters, vegetable acids, and peculiar flavoring principles. Fruits and vegetables add a certain bulk to the meal which seems to favor digestion.

Dried fruits, as raisins, figs, etc., have a nutritive value nearly equal to that of bread, containing forty to fifty per cent. of sugar. Raisins have proved an excellent food for Arctic expeditions, sustaining the animal heat under extreme conditions. The importance of this food material may be seen from a statement of the amount prepared in California alone in 1884, viz.: of prunes, 1,870,000 pounds; of apples, 1,600,000; of peaches, 550,000; of sun-dried grapes, 150,000. In 1889 San Diego county alone furnished 150,000 boxes of raisins; while the yield of figs in California the same year was 11,190,816 pounds.

Jellies are a sort of dried fruit-juice. Many fruits contain a substance called *pectin* or *pectose*, which forms when heated with sugar a gelatinous mass which will keep good for a long time if put in a cool and dry place. For a detailed account of the various substances here referred to, see " Food," by A. H. Church.

Since putrefactive fermentation requires germs, moisture, and warmth for its progress, the decay of food substances may be prevented —

(1.) By subjecting them to extremes of temperature: to freezing, so that the germs cannot grow; or to heat equal to or above that of boiling water, so that the germs are killed.

(2.) By the exclusion of germ-laden air, as in

canning or bottling, or by coating the sterile substances with an impervious layer.

(3.) By the removal of moisture, as in drying meats and fruits; vegetables are now so prepared for soups, etc.

(4.) By cooking in concentrated sugar syrup, as in preserves. This combines the removal of moisture with an impervious coating.

There is also the less wholesome, but very common method of preservation by the application of antiseptics : such as salt and smoke for meats ; brandy, vinegar, etc., for fruits ; borax and salicylic acid for various substances. These preparations cannot be as healthful, even if the antiseptic has no direct influence upon the digestive organs, and they should be used sparingly.

NOTE. — The practice of delaying decay by means of cold storage has greatly increased since 1886, so that nearly all articles of food are transported and kept in stock, notably meat, butter, and fruits. By this means the markets are enabled to offer nearly the same variety the year round, and customers, yielding to temptation, buy without much regard to delicacy of flavor and without considering the fact that whatsoever comes out of the cold storage should be either cooked or used before it becomes warm.

It is a well-established fact that cold of this moderate degree does not *prevent* bacterial life, but only *retards* it, and moreover seems to favor a great activity as soon as the cold is removed. Thus creamery butter often becomes almost uneatable within two days after taking from the cold storage.

IX.

OTHER MATERIALS USED IN COOKING.

SINCE light sweet bread is one of the most important articles of diet, and since in the United States such bread is largely made in homes, and not in bakeries, as is the case in Europe, the substances which produce this digestible food deserve consideration.

YEAST.

Yeast is a cryptogamous plant, a simple cell which grows, by multiplication or budding, in a slightly sweetened liquid, converting the sugar into carbonic acid gas and alcohol, at the same time that it acts upon starch, converting it into dextrine, and then into starch sugar. The process is technically called alcoholic *fermentation*, and yeast a *ferment*. Different kinds of fermentation are distinguished by the name of the principal product to which they give rise; as, alcoholic or yeast fermentation, acetic or vinegar fermentation, lactic, butyric, etc.

It is because of the evolution of carbonic acid gas, which is held in the sponge in little bubbles by the tenacity of the gluten of the wheat, that yeast is used in the preparation of bread. Wild yeast germs are floating in the air, and the leaven of olden times owed its efficiency to the cells which fell into the open vessel. The objection to this spontaneous fermentation is, that not only the cells of alcoholic fermentation fall in, but those that produce the other kinds, notably the lactic, so that bread-making by leaven is a somewhat haphazard process: the result may be fairly good, and it may be very bad. The black sour bread of Germany and other European countries is made in this manner. The addition of hops retards decay of the yeast. Modern yeast is brewers' or beer yeast, even home-made preparations being mostly started by it; because both for beer and bread the alcoholic fermentation is desirable, and brewers, by careful study and experiment, have learned so to control the process as to obtain a yeast consisting of only one kind of organisms, *Saccharomyces cerevisiæ*.

When yeast is added to batter, it is like the scattering of a multitude of little living cells or seeds, ready to grow with extraordinary rapidity in a medium suited to their nutrition. These cells, in well mixed batter, are present at every point, and as each cell, in decomposing sugar, gives off tiny bubbles of carbonic acid gas, these bubbles are in every part of the dough, rendering it porous or "light." Although wheat flour contains only about one per cent of sugar, when fermentation is once started, the starch is rapidly converted into sugar, and the sugar so formed into carbonic acid gas and alcohol : thus the fermentation of bread goes on at the expense of the starch of the flour. Cooked starch is acted on more readily than raw, and therefore the addition of some boiled potatoes to the sponge causes a more rapid rising.

There are two divisions of beer yeast, high (*haute*) and low (*basse*). According to Pasteur the *high* buds more rapidly, floats, and is produced by fermentation at from fifty to seventy-five degrees Fahrenheit. The *low* sinks, the cells are more separate, it buds for a short time only, and is produced at a lower temperature, forty to fifty degrees, and is of late much used for beer. The best yeast for bread is that which floats. It is now prepared for the purpose, and when ready for use is skimmed off, drained, pressed in sacks, cut up into squares, covered with tin-foil, and sold as compressed yeast. In this condition it is next best to the fresh brewers' yeast, with the advantage of small bulk and ease of transportation. If kept cool and dry, it will be good for days; and if dried, not in the sun or in the oven, but in a current of warm air, it will keep indefinitely. Packages of dry yeast are composed for the most part of yeast mixed with corn or rye meal and then dried. Yeast germs are killed by a temperature of boiling water, and freezing arrests their growth. The best temperature for fermentation of beer yeast is from sixty to seventy degrees Fahrenheit.

Since the sole object of bread fermentation is the production of a porous loaf, Miss Corson's recommendation of the quick process of raising bread in two hours, by the use of two squares of yeast, seems to have a reasonable basis, and if the bread is, as it should be, well baked, so that the inside of the loaf has reached a temperature of boiling water, there will remain no yeasty flavor. Many loaves do not become heated to this point even when burned on the outside, consequently the yeast germs are not killed: such slack-baked bread is not wholesome.

Yeast is not often adulterated, but its quality may

vary owing to carelessness in preparation, especially if it is home-made. There is no doubt that the compressed or Vienna yeast is the best article now at hand for producing the so-called raised bread. The color of good yeast is yellow or grayish yellow; the browner its tint, the more dead germs there are. It should be only a mass of cells with no fibre or tissue. Occasionally a blue line is seen : this is due to the presence of *Mucors*, or moulds. Such yeast makes bread which will become mouldy in a very short time.

The following notes of the microscopic appearances of yeast may be useful. Take some yeast on the point of a pin, and add carefully a drop of water on the slide. Cover and examine with reflected light under a power of six hundred diameters. The cells are seen not to be round, but rather oval, a little pointed at each end : the larger they are, the better the yeast. The walls are transparent and delicate, to allow of ready osmosis. The contents of new cells are clear, limpid, and colorless, somewhat granulated with one or more vacuoles. Old cells have darker contents, are more coarsely granulated, and destitute of vacuoles, they are of irregular form and look withered. Strange ferments are almost always encountered as impurities. *Saccha-*

romyces exiguus, or *minor*, is often abundant, if the fermentation which produced the yeast was carried on at a low temperature. It is about half the size of *S. cerevisiæ*, or only three ten-thousandths of an inch in diameter, and is always present in leaven. *Penicillium glaucum*, *Mucor mucedo*, or Mould, etc., may be readily recognized. There may be present *micrococci*, or round cells, and *bacilli*, or rod-like cells, giving rise to various other fermentations, all of which soon pass over into the putrid fermentation: the time elapsing varies according to the temperature, etc.

"On Fermentation," by Schützenberger, and "Études sur la Bière," by Pasteur, are books to be consulted. Dr. Graham's "Chemistry of Bread-Making" is a valuable addition to the literature of the subject.

SODA, BAKING-POWDERS, ETC.

The problem of making porous bread without the long process of fermentation, and the consequent loss in material which is converted into carbonic acid and alcohol, has often occupied the thought of chemists of reputation. The results have been: —

First, aerated bread, made by forcing into the dough,

just before baking, carbonic acid gas prepared by chemical means in another vessel.

Secondly, the so-called soda bread of this country, in which the carbonic acid gas is liberated from bicarbonate of soda by the use of an acid; as muriatic, tartaric, lactic (sour milk), and the acid tartrate of potassium (cream of tartar), acid phosphate of calcium, or acid lactate of calcium.

Thirdly, baking-powder bread, which is now (1898) almost universally used in the United States in place of soda bread. The great advantage to the community is, that while baking-powders are composed of the same materials as those mentioned above, they are carefully mixed, so that neither acid nor alkali shall be in excess.

Soda (bicarbonate, supercarbonate, or cooking soda) is chemically a sodium hydrogen carbonate prepared by subjecting recrystallized sal soda, or washing soda, to an atmosphere of carbonic acid gas. The only impurities likely to be found are some sulphates and chlorides remaining from the process of manufacture of the sal soda. The substances used to liberate the carbonic acid gas are practically reduced to two, *cream of tartar*, and *acid phosphate of calcium*. The first is prepared from imported argols, a substance used by calico printers and dyers. It is the crust which is formed on wine casks in the process of fermentation. In its refined and purified condition it is sold for bread-making. One baking-powder manufactory, at least, is said to use only that which has been chemically prepared. The price being from forty to eighty cents per pound, and in times of disturbance of foreign commerce even twice that, cream of tartar is the most liable to be adulterated of all the articles used in cooking.

Terra alba, sulphate of calcium, or, as it is commonly called, *gypsum*, is the substance most frequently used to make up ten to ninety per cent of the weight of cream of tartar. It is reported that fine bone-ash has been found in some samples from the Western States. In Eastern Massachusetts the most frequent adulterant is the much cheaper acid phosphate of calcium; and since this is itself used as a substitute for cream of tartar, the effect on the bread is not as much to be feared as if gypsum were used. If it shall be proved that a certain amount of potassium salts are desirable to counteract the excessive use of salt and salted foods, the much discussed cream of tartar bread may find its place as a recognized article of diet.

Acid phosphate of calcium is prepared from bones by treating them with sulphuric acid, setting free a portion of the phosphoric acid. It is supposed to be a useful ingredient of bread, since it restores some of the phosphate said to be lost in the bran.

Acid lactate of calcium has lately been used for a cream of tartar substitute, and in many respects it promises well. It contains the same acid as sour milk, and is prepared from starch by the action of the lactic ferment.

Baking Powders, prepared from soda and cream of tartar chiefly, are, when put up in tin cans, with the maker's name on the label, much more reliable than any other form of bread-raising preparation. About eighty per cent are found to be good; of cream of tartar only sixty per cent are genuine. Sometimes a very little bicarbonate of ammonia is added, to secure a complete neutralization of the acid without leaving an excess of soda. If this amount does not exceed one per cent, it can do no harm. As they are made in large quantities, they are of a more even composition than when cooks guess at the proportions by spoonfuls. The chief adulterant used is starch or rice flour, sometimes to the extent of fifty per cent. There is not so much adulteration as has often been supposed, if the articles are purchased of the large firms and of reliable dealers. Alum is not infrequently found in powders sold in bulk. The following simple tests may be of use to those who have had a little practice in chemistry.

Good cream of tartar is soluble in eighteen parts of boiling water. Good baking powder is also soluble; a small quantity of starch present will give a certain opacity to the solution, but if in excess a paste may be formed stiff enough for laundry use. If there is in either case much residue insoluble in water which dissolves in hydrochloric acid, phosphate or sulphate of calcium is to be suspected.

A few drops of barium chloride added to the hydrochloric acid solution will cause a white precipitate, if sulphates are present in the substance under examination. If the phosphates are to be tested for, the acid to be used for a solution is nitric, and to the solution a few cubic centimeters of molybdate of ammonia are added. A fine yellow color or precipitate indicates phosphates. Ammonia is sometimes found in baking powders. If present, a small lump of potassium hydrate added to the strong aqueous solution will, on heating, cause the ammonia to be given off in the steam, which will then turn red litmus-paper blue.

To test for alum, prepare a fresh decoction of logwood; add a few drops to the solution or substance, and render it acid by acetic acid. A yellow color proves the absence of alum; a purplish red or a bluish color, more or less decided, means more or less alum. If the substance were not acidified, the test might be vitiated by the presence of an alkali, as in the case of a baking powder. Caution: use a new solution, or a new portion of an old one, for each test.

To judge of the quantity of any of the substances, it is necessary to have a standard article with which to compare the suspected one. If the same quantity of each is taken, and it is subjected to the same tests, a very correct judgment of its quality may be formed. Acids should be used in glass or china vessels only.

X.

PRINCIPLES OF DIET.

THE food of savage and semi-civilized man has always been of the material most readily obtained; either the flesh of animals killed in the chase, or wild fruits native to his country, or the products of crude agriculture.[1] The nations of Northern Europe, down to nearly the middle of the present century, ate rye and barley bread, as wheat could not be profitably grown in that region; and the Esquimaux to-day live upon the product of the seal fishery from necessity, and not from choice.

Now, the food products of the whole world are accessible to the people of the United States, through the use of improved methods of transportation, — the refrigerator car and steamship compartment, — and through improved methods of preservation, by cold storage, and by the canning process.

---

[1] For the diet of ancient peoples, see "Food and Dietetics," Pavy, p. 475.

This very abundance brings its own danger; for the appetite is no longer a sufficient guide to the selection of food, as it was in the case of the early peoples who were not tempted by so great a variety.

Many diseases of modern civilization are doubtless due to errors of diet, which might easily be avoided. Many dietaries have been published, but nearly all are only of limited local application, so that, when applied elsewhere, they have failed, and brought discredit upon the whole plan. Only certain broad principles can be laid down, and much intelligent study must be brought to bear upon the question in each community.

The first general principle is suggested by Dr. Pavy, when he calls attention to the fact that the meat-eaters among animals, having to hunt for their food, pass long intervals without any, and when it is obtained gorge themselves with it, and then lie torpid for days. The herbivorous animals, having their food always near them, eat all the time, and are stupid all the time.

Man ought not to imitate either class. It is his privilege to choose such times of eating and such materials for food as will best develop his mental power. Many writers seem to forget this, and to plan man's food as if he were a mere animal, whereas he is or may be very much more. His food should be such as to keep the animal mechanism in good order for the mind to use. It should not be overfed, so as to be sluggish, nor should it be starved, so as to be incapable of executing the mind's demands. The chief office of the food, then, is to preserve health.

Each person born into the world has certain work to do, and, to do the work, energy or force is required. The only source of human energy is the food. The wrong kind of food, and either too much or too little in quantity, means work undone or energy wasted. This is the second principle of diet. The third general principle is an economical one. In spite of the seeming abundance of the country, the average value of our produce, if distributed *per capita*, would be only from 40 to 45 cents per day, out of which shelter, food, and clothing must be provided. Statistics show that the mere price of food constitutes 60 per cent. of the cost of living of the working people of the United States, and it may well be said that "half the struggle of life is a struggle for food for the large majority of people." To quote Professor

Atwater:[1] "The average person selects the different food materials with less knowledge of their actual value (as a source of nourishment) than is found in almost any other line of purchases."

In view of these facts the study of dietaries should be undertaken by intelligent housewives, by students of domestic science and household economics, as well as by the governments of cities, States, and countries. The simple underlying principles of nutrition and dietary work should be taught in the schools in connection with the cookery.

The U. S. Government has conducted many of these dietary studies, from which reliable data may be obtained concerning "the food economy of people in different parts of the country and under different conditions of age, sex, health, occupation, and environment."

The general plan of such investigations includes an account of the amounts and composition of all food materials in the house at the beginning, purchased during, and remaining at the end of the period of the investigation, and, when practicable, of all the kitchen and table wastes. The amount of different

[1] "Dietary Studies in N. Y. City in 1895 and 1896."

food materials on hand at the beginning and received during the period are added together; from their sum the amounts remaining at the end are subtracted. This gives the amount of each material actually used. From the amount thus obtained and the composition of each material, as shown by analysis, the amounts of the nutritive ingredients are estimated. From these are subtracted the amounts of nutrients in the waste, and thus the amounts of nutrients actually eaten are learned.

As the result of investigations in the science of nutrition, and from actual study of American dietaries, the following standards are, at present, accepted, although they differ from those formerly proposed by Voit and others in Europe.

It has been estimated that a growing person needs four times as much fat and carbohydrate as of proteid food, while for a grown person the proportion is one of proteid to five or six of carbohydrate.

From this a ration may be computed sufficient to sustain life without work:

Proteid.	Fat.	Carbohydrates.
75 grams,	40 grams,	325 grams,
or	or	or
2.6 oz.	1.7 oz.	11.4 oz.

For an average daily work ration is given:

Proteid.	Fat.	Carbohydrates.
125 grams,	125 grams,	450 grams,
or	or	or
4.4 oz.	4.4 oz.	15.8 oz.

For hard manual labor this latter ration should be increased by one-third.

These weights represent the average amounts of dry and pure food needed daily for each man — the standard being a man weighing 156 pounds.

For a woman and for each child from thirteen to sixteen years eight-tenths of the above rations should be allowed, and for children under ten years an average of five-tenths is reckoned.

In nearly all food materials there is a portion, more or less large, which in preparation or in digestion is not made available for the needs of the body. This waste for all kinds of food averages about ten per cent. The amount of food bought must, then, contain ten per cent. more than the weights of the above rations.

Two questions now present themselves:

1. What might furnish this daily ration, if the science of nutrition could be made a part of the common knowledge?

2. How much could the cost be reduced and the nutritious properties increased at the same time?

Answers to these questions may be found in the following rations selected from many tables, computed with great pains by Professor Atwater and his assistant, Mr. Rockwood, from analyses made for the Smithsonian Institution.

	Cents.
Liver, ½ lb.	5.00
Potatoes, 1 lb.	1.00
Butter, 1 oz.	2.00
Corn Meal, 1 lb.	3.00
Bread, ½ lb.	3.00
	14.00
Beef, Shin, ¼ lb.	1.50
Fresh Cod, ½ lb.	4.00
Oatmeal, ⅛ lb.	.50
Bread, ½ lb.	3.00
Potatoes, 1 lb.	1.00
Milk, ½ pt.	1.50
Corn Meal, ½ lb.	1.50
Butter, 1 oz.	2.00
Boston Crackers, 2 oz.	1.25
	16.25
Round Steak, ½ lb.	8.00
Milk ½ lb.	2.00
Bread, ½ lb.	2.50
Potatoes, 1½ lb.	1.50
Turnips, ½ lb.	.50
Corn Meal, ⅓ lb.	1.00
Butter, 1 oz.	2.00
Cheese, 1 oz.	1.00
Sugar, 1½ oz.	1.00
	19.50
Soda Crackers, ¼ lb.	2.50
Potatoes, 1 lb.	1.00
Bread ½ lb.	3.00
Shad ¼ lb.	4.00
Eggs, ¼ lb.	4.00
Oatmeal, ⅛ lb.	.625
Rice, ⅛ lb.	1.50

	Cents.
Sugar, ⅛ lb.	1.25
Butter, 1 oz.	2.00
Beans, ¼ lb.	1.50
	21.375
Oyster Crackers, ¼ lb.	3.00
Oysters, ½ lb.	10.00
Mutton, Leg, ¼ lb.	4.00
Pease, ⅛ lb.	1.25
Potatoes, 1 lb.	1.00
Oatmeal, ¼ lb.	1.00
Rice, ¼ lb.	2.50
Bread, ½ lb.	3.00
Butter, 1½ oz.	3.00
	28.75
Turkey, ¼ lb.	18.00
Fresh Pork, 2 oz.	1.625
Hominy, ½ lb.	2.00
Potatoes, 1 lb.	1.00
Beans, ¼ lb.	1.50
Rye Bread, ½ lb.	3.00
Milk, 1 lb.	3.50
	30.625
Salmon, ¼ lb.	10.00
Beef, Sirloin, ¼ lb.	5.00
Oysters, ½ lb.	10.00
Dried Beef, 1 oz.	1.00
Wheat Bread, ¼ lb.	3.00
Oatmeal, 2 oz.	.625
Rice, 2 oz.	1.50
Potatoes, ½ lb.	.50
Sweet Potatoes, 1 lb.	6.00
Cabbage, 2 oz.	.25

Turnips, 2 oz.	.125
Butter, 2 oz.	2.00
Milk, 1 lb.	3.50
Sugar, 2 oz.	1.50
	45.00

The following table is given simply as an indication of the kind of calculation which every cooking class should undertake, and which every philanthropist interested in the better living of the people should study. The subject is yet in its infancy, and there is much work to be done in this line before the working people can be well fed at a low cost.

Amount of Nutrients furnished for Twenty-five Cents in Food Materials at ordinary Prices.

Food Materials.	At Prices in Cents per lb.	Twenty-five Cents will pay for lbs.	Containing Nutrients in lbs.
Oysters at 50 cts. per qt.	25	1.00	.12
Oysters at 35 cts. per qt.	17.5	1.42	.17
Bluefish	10	2.50	.27
Beef Sirloin	25	1.00	.29
Shad	12	2.08	.29
Cod	8	3.13	.34
Mutton, Leg	22	1.14	.34
Mackerel	10	2.50	.35
Beef, Round	18	1.39	.40
Canned Salmon	20	1.25	.44
Mutton, Side	20	1.25	.46
Beef, Round	15	1.67	.49

Salt Mackerel	12.5	2.00	.60
Butter	30	0.83	.73
Milk at 8 cts. per qt.	4	6.25	.74
Salt Cod	5	5.00	.82
Milk at 7 cts. per qt.	3.5	7.14	.84
Cheese, whole milk	15	1.67	1.08
Smoked Herring	6	4.17	1.21
Pork, salted, fat	12	2.08	1.65
Wheat Bread	6	4.17	2.75
Potatoes at $1 per bushel	1.7	13.24	3.04
Beans at 10 cts. per qt.	5	5.00	3.96
Potatoes at 75 cts. per bushel	1.25	18.00	4.13
Wheat Bread	4	6.25	4.15
Oatmeal	5	5.00	4.48
Wheat Flour	4	6.25	5.44
Potatoes, 50 cts. per bushel	0.85	26.47	6.06
Indian Meal	3	8.33	6.90

"It is well worth noting that oatmeal is one of the cheapest foods that we have: that is, it furnishes more nutritive material in proportion to the cost than almost any other. Corn meal is indeed cheaper, but the oatmeal has this great advantage over corn meal and wheat flour, that it has more protein. If one wishes to economize in his food, oatmeal rightly cooked affords an excellent material therefor."

It must be remembered, however, that the chemist is not always a cook, or even a physiologist, and that, while a certain combination may look to be very nutritious on paper, it may not prove satisfactory in practice; for the important factor of palatability is left out, and however nutritious a food may be, if it is repulsive to the individual the secretion of the digestive fluids will not follow its ingestion. The art of cookery must here come to the rescue; also the relative digestibility of food must be considered. Nevertheless, calculations such as the preceding are very useful, and worthy of careful study, as indicating a possible economy of the precious food materials.

LIST OF WORKS CONSULTED.

Food. A. H. Church. London, Chapman and Hall, 1882.

Foods. Edward Smith. 8th edition. London, Kegan Paul, Trench, & Co., 1883.

Food and Dietetics. F. W. Pavy. 2d edition. London, Churchill, 1875.

Food and Feeding. Sir Henry Thompson. 3d edition. London, Warne & Co.

The Chemistry of Cookery. W. Mathieu Williams. New York, Appleton & Co., 1885.

The Chemistry of Cooking and Cleaning. Ellen H. Richards and S. Maria Elliott. Boston, Home Science Pub. Co., 1897.

Water Supply. Chemical and Sanitary. Wm. Ripley Nichols. New York, John Wiley and Sons, 1883.

International Health Exhibition Handbooks. — On Food and Food Adjuncts. Diet in Relation to Health and Work. A. Wynter Blyth. — Water, Water Supplies, and Unfermented Beverages. John Attfield. — Principles of Cooking. Septimus Berdmore. — Food and Cooking for Infants. Catherine Jane Wood. — English and Exotic Fruits. W. T. Thisleton Dyer. — Salt and other Condiments. J. J. Manley. — London, Wm. Clowes and Sons, 1884. One shilling each.

Familiar Lessons on Food and Nutrition. T. Twining. London, David Bogue, 1882.

The Chemistry of Bread Making. Charles Graham. Cantor Lectures, London Society of Arts, 1880.

Coffee and Tea. G. V. Poore. London, Lewis, 1883.
What the Grocers sell Us. P. H. Felker. New York, Orange Judd & Co., 1880.
Massachusetts State Board of Health Reports, Papers in. Boston, 1870 to 1884, especially 1879 and 1880-83.
New York State Board of Health Reports, Papers in. 1882-83.
Various Papers by W. O. Atwater. Middletown, Conn.
The Application of Science to the Production and Consumption of Food. Edward Atkinson. Salem, Mass., Press of the A. A. A. S.
The Science of Nutrition. Edward Atkinson, 1892. Damrell & Upham, Boston.
Foods. Their Composition and Analysis. A. Wynter Blyth. London, Griffin & Co., 1882.
Food. Its Adulterations and the Methods for their Detection. Arthur Hill Hassall. London, Longmans, Green, & Co., 1876.
The Analysis and Adulteration of Foods. Parts I. and II. James Bell. London, Chapman and Hall, 1881.
The Microorganisms of Fermentation. Alfred Jörgensen, 1889. F. W. Lyon, London.
Die menschlichen Nahrungs- und Genussmittel. Dr. J. König. 2d edition. Berlin, Julius Springer, 1883. 2 vols.
Die wichtigsten Nahrungsmittel und Getränke. Oscar Dietzsch. 4th edition. Zurich, 1884.
Praxis des Nahrungsmittel Chemikers. F. Elsner. Leipzig, 1880.
Studien über den chemischen Nachweis fremder Fette in Butterfette. Dr. August Hannsen. Erlangen, 1884. Pamphlet.
Butter, its Analysis and Adulteration. Hehner and Angell. London, Churchill, 1877.
Water Analysis. Dr. E. Frankland. London, 1880.

No. 46. Dietary Studies in New York City, 1895-1896.
No. 43. Losses in Boiling Vegetables, and the Composition and Digestibility of Potatoes and Eggs.
No. 28. The Chemical Composition of American Food Materials.
No. 34. The Carbohydrates of Wheat, Maize, Flour, and Bread, etc.
No. 48. Zinc in Evaporated Apples.
No. 25. Dairy Bacteriology.
No. 44. Preliminary Investigations on the Metabolism of Nitrogen and Carbon in the Human Organism.
No. 54. Nutrition Investigations in New Mexico in 1898.

Bureau of Annual Industry. Circulars:
11. How to Select Good Cheese.

INDEX.

	PAGE
Acid Lactate	159
Phosphate	157, 159
Acids in Fruits	147
in Vinegar	141
Adulteration	18, 20, 22, 73
of baking powder	160
of butter	95
of cayenne pepper	130
of cheese	96
of cocoa	68
of coffee	64
of cream of tartar	160
of flour	84
of honey	117
of milk	89
of mustard	127
of pepper	129
of spices	131
of sugar	113
of tea	154
of vinegar	141
Aerated Bread	156
Alchemist, the modern	20
Allspice	134
Antiseptics	150
Arrowroot	87
Bacteria	29
Baking Powder	157, 159
Barley	72
Beans	146

	PAGE
Beet-root Sugar	102
Block-tin Pipes	45
Books of Reference	177
Bread	151
Buckwheat	86
Butter	89, 91
Caffeine	62
Canned Fruits and Meats	118
rules for soundness of	124
Cassia	133
Cayenne Pepper	130
Cereal Foods	70
Cheese	95
Chocolate	67
Cider	141
Cinnamon	132
Cloves	134
Cocoa	67
Coffee	59
Cooks, educated	11, 168
Corn Meal	16, 173
Corn Starch	87
Cost of Daily Ration	165, 174, 175
Cream	91
Cream of Tartar	20, 21, 23, 157
Currants	147
Curry	135
Daily Ration	165
Decay of Food	149

INDEX.

	PAGE
Diet, articles of	16, 162
Dietaries	165
Disease and drinking water	25, 27, 31, 35
Dried Fruits	148
Economy, domestic	14, 15, 17, 168
Ergot	76
Extracts, Flavoring	139
Farina	87
Fehling's Solution	115
Fermentation	90, 140, 151
putrefactive	149, 156
Filtration of water	35, 37
Fish	145
Flour	71, 78, 80
Fruits	147
Germs	30, 149, 152
Germ Theory	29
Ginger	135
Glucose	97, 104, 106, 112
Gluten	85
Grape Sugar	103
Gypsum	23, 158
Hardness of water	26, 40
Honey	107, 113, 117
Housekeeping, as a profession	10
scientific	16
Iron Pipes	46
Jellies	149
Lead in canned foods	122
Pipes	41
Leaven	152
Lentils	146
Macaroni	87
Mace	133
Maize	75
Maple Sugar	103
Meat	144

	PAGE
Milk	22, 88
Condensed	90
disease carried by	31
Millet	75
Molassess	99, 104
Mustard	125
Nutmegs	131
Oatmeal	74, 173
Oats	74
Oil, salad	138
Oleomargarine	94
Peas	146
Pepper	128
Pickles	142
Pimento	134
Poisons	32
Pollution of Wells	35
Price of Food	164, 172
Raisins	149
Relishes	148
Rice	73
Rye	76
Salt	143
Samovar	57
Shells, Cocoa	68
Soda	157
Soft Water	26
Softening of hard Water	39
Spices	130
Starch	86, 153
Starch Sugar	106
Sugar	97
Sucrose	97, 104
Syrup	100, 116
Tables of Rations	169
Tables of Cost of Food	172
Tannin	51, 62, 67
Tea	49

INDEX.

	PAGE		PAGE
Terra Alba	158	Vinegar	139
Theine	51	Water	24
Tin Cans	118	suitable for domestic use	32
in food	119	Wells	35
		Wheat	76
Utility, law of	14	Wheat Flour, grinding of	78
Vegetables	147	Yeast	151
Vermicelli	87	microscopic examination of	155

www.ingramcontent.com/pod-product-compliance
Lightning Source LLC
Chambersburg PA
CBHW020247170426
43202CB00008B/268